Nursing Homes and Nursing Care

Lessons from the Teaching Nursing Homes

Mathy D. Mezey, R.N., Ph.D., F.A.A.N. is Professor of Gerontological Nursing, Associate Director Ralston-Penn Center for Care, Education, and Research for the Aged, School of Nursing, University of Pennsylvania in Philadelphia. She has a long-standing involvement in the preparation of nurses to work with the elderly. Her research has focused on assessment and the response of older patients following a hip fracture. She is the former Director of the Robert Wood Johnson Foundation Teaching Nursing Home Program.

Joan E. Lynaugh, R.N., Ph.D., F.A.A.N. is Associate Professor, Director of the Center for the Study of the History of Nursing, School of Nursing, University of Pennsylvania in Philadelphia. Her research interests are concentrated in contemporary health care delivery and the history of health care in the United States. She is the former Associate Director of the Robert Wood Johnson Foundation Teaching Nursing Home Program.

Mary M. Cartier is the former Assistant Program Director of the Robert Wood Johnson Foundation Teaching Nursing Home Program and Associate Director of the Johnson Regional Consultative Conferences. She is currently Executive Assistant to the Dean, School of Arts and Sciences, University of Pennsylvania, Philadelphia.

Nursing Homes and Nursing Care

Lessons from the Teaching Nursing Homes

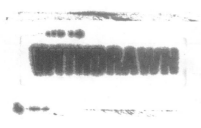

Mathy D. Mezey
R.N., Ph.D., F.A.A.N.
Joan E. Lynaugh
R.N., Ph.D., F.A.A.N.
Mary M. Cartier
Editors

SPRINGER PUBLISHING COMPANY
NEW YORK

Springer Publishing Company, Inc.
536 Broadway
New York, NY 10012

89 90 91 92 93 / 5 4 3 2 1

Library of Congress Cataloging in Publication Data

Nursing homes and nursing care.

   Based on a six-year experiment with the Robert Wood
Johnson Foundation's Teaching Nursing Home Program.
   Includes bibliographies and index.
   1. Teaching nursing homes—United States.
2. Geriatric nursing.   I. Mezey, Mathy Doval.
II. Lynaugh, Joan E.   III. Cartier, Mary M.   IV. Teach-
ing Nursing Home Program.   [DNLM: 1. Education, Nursing.
2. Geriatric Nursing.   3. Nursing Care—standards—
United States.   4. Nursing Homes—United States.
WY 152 N974608]
RA997.N895   1988   610.73'3'071   88-30102
ISBN 0-8261-6210-X

Printed in the United States of America

Contents

v

Foreword

This book is an account of an experiment in mutual trust, an experiment in geriatric nursing—an experiment that worked.

I first heard the term "geriatric nursing" in 1947. I was one of a group of young nurses, recently discharged after service in World War II, who met with Mary Roberts, editor of the *American Journal of Nursing*, to seek her advice on our careers. "Geriatric nursing," she told us, "was about to become important." It was only after we consulted a dictionary that we learned the word "geriatric" referred to care for the aged. I still remember that moment of discovery 40 years later.

The term "geriatric nursing" may be relatively new but the concept is not. Nurses were caring for elderly patients in the hospital or in the home from the earliest days of the profession. Over time, "old people's care" became a kind of subspecialty in nursing, one not particularly known for its intellectual challenge or professional preparation but rather one that required kindness, patience, and a strong back.

Nursing, as with all professions, expresses its philosophy and content through its literature as well as its educational programs and practice. That nursing was concerned with the older patient is evident from the nearly 700 articles on the health of the elderly published in nursing journals between 1956 and 1968. That the literature of the day revealed an enormous disparity between what was known and what was practiced is evident from the cheery anecdotal tone of such representative articles as "The elderly can be happy," "Our task can be done better," and "We succeeded in keeping patients out of bed."

But in the late 1960s and through the 1970s, as the American population began to age more rapidly and new career opportunities opened up for women, the nursing profession soon found that kindness, patience, and a strong back, while useful, were simply not enough to meet the needs of the growing numbers of frail and dependent elderly. New nursing research on the care of the aged began to be reported and geriatric nursing took on new significance as a respected professional subspecialty—gerontological nursing.

Unfortunately, the growing body of gerontological research did not result in improved nursing practice. With the exception of a few exemplary geriatric institutions, patterns of care for the institutionalized elderly showed little change. Most of the new knowledge was discussed in the classroom, read in the library, but seldom applied in the nursing home. Collaboration between the medical and nursing professions, whether in not-for-profit or for-profit nursing homes, was almost nonexistent.

Nursing home care in the early 1980s showed little improvement. Health professionals whose goal was to "tip the scales in favor of the patient" were frustrated by the continuing disparity between what they knew was possible and what was being done in caring for the aged.

It was at this time a new concept surfaced—the Teaching Nursing Home Program. It was a concept born of an obvious need and professional chagrin that, despite the prediction in the 1940s that "geriatric nursing was about to become important," care of the aged was still a neglected nursing focus.

From the outset, the concept of the Teaching Nursing Home was recognized as a high-risk experiment. The program required that stronger ties be established between outstanding schools of nursing, nurse educators and researchers, and cooperating nursing homes. No data existed that would support the likelihood of its success. On the contrary, many skeptics felt that the required inter- and intra-disciplinary linkages and the enormous effort to put them into play were insurmountable obstacles to the project's success. Fear of change, fear of new costs, and fear of losing autonomy also caused many to back away from the experiment. There were other stumbling blocks. Governmental regulations concerning payment systems had to be considered. And, most importantly, the daily routines of the nursing staffs involved in the program, would be drastically changed.

When the Teaching Nursing Home Program first began in 1982, the nurses who were coordinating the project asked me to serve as a consultant, since I was a retired geriatric nurse with long teaching experience. In this capacity, I looked over the shoulders of those who brought the program to life and those who made it work. I attended each of the national meetings, witnessed the program's progress from early discussions of its possibility to the present, and observed each crucial stage in this pioneering experiment.

From the beginning, those who initiated the Teaching Nursing Home Program—the Robert Wood Johnson Foundation which funded it, the University of Pennsylvania faculty who coordinated it, and the American Academy of Nursing which co-sponsored it—recognized that breaking down existing barriers between the caregiving institutions and the academic nursing centers would pose a problem of trust.

In 1981, announcements of the program went out to eligible schools of nursing and service institutions. One hundred and ninety-three responded with a letter of intent to submit a proposal. The "paper planning" at this stage involved the identification of collaborating institutions, preparation of tentative budgets, consideration of contractual arrangements, and preliminary selection of potential key personnel. Attitudes toward the project ranged from enthusiasm to apprehension, but there was general agreement that risks had to be taken. One applicant described this phase as "an attempt to take the head and heart of academic nursing and combine that with the heart and hands of the caring institutions." Those who had expressed an initial interest in the project were invited to a national exploratory preproposal meeting to help them decide whether they wished to pursue their intent to participate.

After careful winnowing of the competitive proposals and 18 site visits, 11 grants were finally funded in 1982. Annual meetings were planned so that representatives of the participating institutions could discuss ideas and problems. The first annual meeting in 1982, as expected, was essentially a discussion of problems. The "doing" which was already underway had yet to produce tangible results, and the mood of the participants was one of guarded hope, tempered by considerable uncertainty.

At the second annual meeting in 1983, there were limited success stories. In many cases, negotiations that had already been successfully completed had to begin all over again because of personnel changes, unforeseen obstacles, or on-site changes in management or medical staff. Medicare changes altered the patient populations. Nevertheless, the participants had grown to trust one another and delegates at this meeting freely and openly discussed their experiences concerning "what had worked" and "what had failed." Not only a wide range of ideas but also a few publications were beginning to emerge.

By the third annual meeting in 1984, a dramatic change was noted. The participants were in control of events, able to plan collaboratively and able to face those disasters which still occurred at times. This meeting was a high point in the five-year project. Colleagues from all 11 programs taught and learned from one another. Reports and workshop sessions were complemented by nonstop informal discussions that ranged from the friendly exchange of concepts and practical suggestions to mutual support. Above all, people had learned to trust themselves. No fourth annual meeting was needed—everyone was too busy with the local projects. The *Teaching Nursing Home Newsletter* and a growing number of Teaching Nursing Home publications in the nursing literature kept communication open among the participating agencies.

At the closing meeting in 1987, a 200-person Invitational Conference, participants faced a new issue: How do we pass on what we have learned? How can this experimental program, with its attendant risks, joys, and pains, tip the scales in favor of quality care for nursing home patients across the country?

This book will help point the way, for it summarizes what we have learned from a six-year experiment in social change, an experiment in mutual trust: the Teaching Nursing Home.

DORIS SCHWARTZ, R.N., F.A.A.N.

Preface

In 1981 The Robert Wood Johnson Foundation (RWJF) initiated the Teaching Nursing Home Program (TNHP) to serve as a catalyst to improve care in nursing homes. The underlying assumption was that involving nursing schools and, more specifically, introducing highly skilled nurses into nursing homes would significantly improve standards of patient care, help recruit and retain clinical staff, and more effectively use nurse and physician services in the care of nursing home patients.

A national invitational conference marking the end of the TNHP, held in Philadelphia in 1987, provided an opportunity to reflect on the origins, accomplishments, and implications of this experiment in social change. The papers presented at this conference and the discussion they generated highlighted the fact that the TNHP had very different meanings for different people. Linda Aiken, as Vice President at the RWJF, conceived of the program in 1980 at a time of nursing home crisis and prior to the implementation of prospective payment. From 1981, program staff at the University of Pennsylvania guided the 11 sites. Faculty and nursing home staff implemented, molded, and at times rejected program goals. Evaluators now wrestle with assessment of the program outcomes. And, in their roles as armchair quarterbacks, outside observers offer opinions as to the program's effectiveness or lack thereof. In this book the authors illustrate the many thoughts expressed at the conference and give voice to the TNHP's various themes.

The first, and perhaps most important, theme is the special idea or model of care found in a good nursing home. This theme is expressed by many of the authors—in Doris Schwartz's foreword, in the chapter by Rosemary Stevens (Chapter 7), and especially in the four case studies in Chapter 6. Robert Heyssel writes about achieving a "state of mind" that is right for nursing home practice, while Carol Lindeman writes about the very different model of care applied by faculty interested in nursing home practice as opposed to hospital practice. Rosemary Stevens refers to the necessity for making and preserving a "conceptual break with the medical mystique," and William Kissick and Karen Knibbe write about participant care, where patients are passengers, constituents, or stake holders rather than objects upon whom caregivers practice their various skills. These authors repeatedly remind us of the "goodness of fit" between nursing values and orientation and the care of the elderly.

Another important theme of the TNHP is the relationship between physicians and nurses in the nursing home. The complexity of this relationship is due to the proximity of the two parties to the elderly and how authority affects their roles. The physician is not constantly in contract with the patient; the nurse is. In real life, of course, personal relationships between nurses and physicians sometimes overcome failure to construct formal understandings about shared clinical decision making. But relying on personal relationships is not enough. The introduction of the clinical specialist/nurse practitioner into the care setting, as occurred in many of these projects, complements the contributions of the physician and establishes the possibility of far better medical and nursing decisions for the benefit of patients. The authors of the first five chapters and Chapter 10 grapple with how to implement, express, evaluate, and fund this potential partnership.

The TNHP experience has helped to underscore the degree to which nursing homes are essential to the fabric of the American health care system. The Teaching Nursing Homes dispelled the myth that many people are inappropriately placed in nursing homes and laid to rest the presumption that everyone is better off with home rather than nursing home care. This legitimization requires reevaluation of past responses to the nursing home as a clinical site for faculty and students. Hospitals can no longer remain aloof to the quality of care provided in nursing homes just as schools of nursing must include experiences in nursing homes in their curricula. The TNHP was a faculty training project, creating a cadre of committed faculty who are fully realistic as to the exigencies of nursing home practice. Jean Miller, Neville Strumpf, and Sister Lucia Gamroth address the academic issues associated with faculty practice in nursing homes.

The TNHP significantly increased the professional resources now committed to improving patient care. While nursing home staff are at the bedside caring for patients, they can be confident that the people speaking at national meetings, presenting to legislatures, or teaching students know and feel very deeply about their issues. Likewise, while faculty involve themselves in national platforms, and analyze, publish, and present their clinical research, they can be confident that their students are being taught by colleagues who understand vital educational goals. Linda Aiken argues that although adequate health care to the elderly is a "complex and multifaceted challenge" teaching nursing homes "offer promise as one strategy to help nursing homes respond to their rapidly changing environment." The commitment of schools of nursing and nursing homes to achieve this goal together may prove to be the Teaching Nursing Homes' lasting legacy.

Contributors

Linda Aiken, Ph.D., F.A.A.N.
Trustee Professor of Nursing
  and Sociology
University of Pennsylvania
Philadelphia, PA 19104-6096

Sharon Arnold, M.P.H.
RAND Corporation
Santa Monica, CA

Joan Buchanan, Ph.D.
RAND Corporation
Santa Monica, CA

Mary Cartier
Executive Assistant to the Dean
School of Arts and Sciences
University of Pennsylvania
Philadelphia, PA 19104-6377

**Sr. Lucia Gamroth, R.N., M.S.,
  M.P.A.**
Associate Administrator
Benedictine Nursing Center
Mount Angel, OR 97362

Judith Garrard, Ph.D.
School of Public Health
University of Minnesota
1260 May Memorial Building
  (Box 197)
420 Delaware Street, SE
Minneapolis, MN 55455

Robert Heyssel, M.D.
President
Johns Hopkins Hospital
600 North Wolfe Street
Baltimore, MD 21205

Robert L. Kane, M.D.
Dean and Professor
School of Public Health
University of Minnesota
1260 Mayo Memorial Building
  (Box 197)
420 Delaware Street, SE
Minneapolis, MN 55455

Rosalie Kane, D.S.W.
School of Public Health
University of Minnesota
1260 Mayo Memorial Building
  (Box 197)
420 Delaware Street, SE
Minneapolis, MN 55455

Alice Kethley, Ph.D.
Executive Director
Benjamin Rose Institute
500 Hanna Building
1422 Euclid Avenue
Cleveland, OH 44115

William Kissick, M.D.
Professor of Public Health
Professor of Research Medicine
School of Medicine
University of Pennsylvania
225 Nursing Education Building
Philadelphia, PA 19104-6096

Karen K. Knibbe, M.S.N.
School of Nursing
University of Pennsylvania
Philadelphia, PA 19104-6377

**Carol Lindeman, Ph.D.,
F.A.A.N.**
Dean, School of Nursing
Associate Director, Nursing
Service
University of Oregon Health
Sciences Center
Portland, OR 97201

Joan Lynaugh, Ph.D., F.A.A.N.
School of Nursing
University of Pennsylvania
Nursing Education Building
Philadelphia, PA 19104-6096

**Susan McDermott, R.N.,
G.N.P.**
Mountain States Health
Corporation

**Mathy D. Mezey, Ed.D.,
F.A.A.N.**
University of Pennsylvania
Nursing Education Building
School of Nursing
Philadelphia, PA 19104-6096

Jean R. Miller, R.N., Ph.D.
Professor and Associate Dean
for Research
College of Nursing
University of Utah
Assistant Director, Nursing
Practice
University of Utah Hospital
Salt Lake City, UT 84112

Sheila Ryan, Ph.D., R.N.
Dean, School of Nursing
Director, Nursing Practice
University of Rochester
601 Elmwoodd Avenue
Rochester, NY 14642

William J. Scanlon, Ph.D.
Co-Director
Center for Health Policy Study
2233 Wisconsin Avenue, NW,
Suite 525
Washington, DC 20007

Rosemary Stevens, Ph.D.
Professor and Chair
Department of History and
Sociology of Science
University of Pennsylvania
Philadelphia, PA 19104-6310

Neville Strumpf, R.N., Ph.D.
Associate Professor
School of Nursing
University of Pennsylvania
Nursing Education Building
Philadelphia, PA 19104-6096

1

Reordering Values: The Teaching Nursing Home Program

Mathy D. Mezey, Joan E. Lynaugh, and Mary M. Cartier

In the minds of patients, families, and health professionals alike, nursing homes still conjure up almost universally negative images. They are viewed as marginal institutions, the orphans of the health care system, representing the failure of hospitals to cure and families to care. Inheriting the onus of both an almshouse-asylum image and "mom and pop" amateurism, nursing homes risk dismissal as institutions caring for people who cannot do better for themselves. Possibly, it may be whispered, people in nursing homes have brought the stigma of illness and dependence on themselves through poor life habits and poverty. Despite evidence to the contrary, people still believe that nursing home patients have been abandoned by their families, or have social ties too tenuous to offer them care when they reach old age. The social stigma of placement is so strong that some families provide home care for elderly relatives to the point of financial ruin and despite deterioration of the family caregiver's own health. Many patients and families assert that they prefer death to nursing home placement.[1]

From another viewpoint nursing homes are seen as transitional social institutions providing necessary care until current deficiencies in hospitals and home care are corrected. Even health professionals continue to believe that patients are inappropriately placed in nursing homes, and that with adequate social support, the majority of nursing home patients could be managed equally well at home. These stereotypes persist in the face of strong evidence that hospitals, nursing homes, and home care agencies generally provide very different care. In fact present day nursing home care is restricted to only the sickest patients with severe functional and mental limitations.[2]

Moreover, instead of recognizing their essential complementarity, hospital and nursing home personnel seem to sustain an adversarial relationship. When patients are transferred from nursing homes to hospitals, the hospital staff often deride the nursing home staff for providing substandard care and failing to diagnose problems in a timely manner. On the other hand, nursing home staff strongly criticize the hospitals' insistence on treating each admission as a new episode of acute illness, and of failing to maintain patients' functional status adequately.

Thus, for health professionals and nonprofessionals alike, nursing homes are on the margin, functioning at the periphery of public consciousness and isolated from the mainstream of health care. Fundamentally, though, America's problem with nursing homes is that they force us to confront both the ultimate futility of the idea of permanent care and the imperative need for protracted care. As gerontological nursing pioneer Doris Schwartz so powerfully phrases it, "Patients who get better are said to do a great service to their caretakers. . . ." Most of the time, the chronically ill fail to do us that service, and they pay heavily for that omission because they conflict with our enormous need to be successful, to be responsible for their dramatic recovery.

The Robert Wood Johnson Foundation Teaching Nursing Home Program (TNHP), inaugurated in 1982, was a direct response to the serious problems created by our negative view of the place of the nursing home in the American health care system. The Program focused on improving clinical care for the frail elderly, educating health care professionals, and sharing responsibility between schools of nursing and nursing homes. It tested the concept that affiliation between university schools of nursing and nursing homes could enhance care and attract more health professionals to nursing home practice, such that the "teaching nursing home" could become the cornerstone for restructuring the place of the nursing home in American health care.

DEMOGRAPHIC CONTEXT FOR THE TEACHING NURSING HOME

During the five years (1982–87) of the Teaching Nursing Home Program, changing demographics, alterations in health care financing, and findings from several national demonstration projects have, indeed, caused a sweeping reexamination of the role of the nursing home in the delivery of health care.

America's aging population is a demographic reality increasingly influencing the delivery of health care. In 1986, 11.5% of the population (25,000,000 people) were over 65 years of age, an eightfold increase since the beginning of the century. The population over 85 will triple over the next 50 years. Older people use significantly all health care services. They make 6.3 physician visits per year versus 4.7 for the general population. Their visits are twice as likely to center around chronic diseases, and return visits are more likely to occur for the same problem than is true for younger patients.[3]

CLINICAL CARE CONTEXT

The burgeoning number of frail elderly persons and the shift in locations where care is delivered have caused legislators to question the adequacy of care provided in nursing homes. Moreover, as hospital and professional school administrators and clinicians become familiar with nursing homes, they too have voiced concern about the quality of the care nursing homes provide. Despite a climate of extreme cost containment in health care, these concerns are sufficiently grave to have prompted recommendations that improvements in quality of care must take precedence over cost. In 1986, the Institute of Medicine's Committee on Nursing Home Regulation published its recommendations for improving the quality of care in nursing homes.[4] Recommendations to improve nursing services were featured in the Committee's report, including the need for RN administered resident assessment, and the need for each resident to receive high quality care to meet individual physical, mental, and psychosocial needs. This report is expected to form the basis for future legislative and regulatory reform.

No longer "mom and pop" institutions, nursing homes have become larger and are increasingly becoming members of groups of facilities operating under one general authority or ownership. In 1985, over half of all certified beds were operated by proprietary or voluntary chains.[5] This large-size corporate administrative structure may work to facilitate dialogue between hospitals and nursing homes.

Because of closer linkages with hospitals and the diversity of clinical problems exhibited by nursing home patients, medical schools are beginning to seek nursing homes as sites for faculty practice, clinical teaching, and research. Geriatrics is now a recognized medical specialty. With support from the National Institute on Aging, the National Institute for Mental Health and the Veterans Administration, medical schools rotate house officers, fellows, and students through community and Veterans Administration nursing homes.

Elderly patients have already significantly changed the case mix in hospitals. In 1986, Medicare reimbursed over 40% of all hospital care.[6] With the advent in 1985 of Medicare prospective payment for acute care, hospitals expanded inpatient geriatric services and began to seek nursing homes as potential partners in the delivery of health services. Because prospective reimbursement encourages judicious use of hospital resources and early discharge to lower levels of care, nursing homes became attractive options for recuperation or hospice services for the dying. Demonstration projects funded by private foundations, such as The Robert Wood Johnson Foundation Hospital Initiatives in Long-term Care, further encourage closer nursing home and hospital linkages. The swing bed program of the early 1980s allowed rural and small community hospitals to convert unneeded hospital beds to skilled nursing beds, creating, in essence, hospital-based nursing homes, a concept now being tested in many larger urban teaching hospitals.[7]

Nursing home placement is often a predictable life experience in old age. Utilization rates suggest that 1 in 5 people over 65 will spend some time in a home prior to their death. For people over 85, this number is 1 in 3. Restrictions on certificates of need have caused a serious bed shortage in many communities and have changed the character of homes from "old age homes" to institutions serving very sick and disabled elderly. The mean age of patients is 81, and 75% are older than 75. The 46% of patients who have lengths of stay (LOS) of less than one year require intensive nursing and rehabilitation, including the application of sophisticated technology.[8] The remaining 50% of patients need maintenance and sustenance over a long period of time, and will probably be maintained in the home until death occurs. They are considerably more debilitated functionally, socially, and mentally than are the elderly living in the community; two-thirds need help with personal care; one-third are markedly restricted in the use of personal space; 66% have two or more chronic diseases; and more than half show signs and symptoms of mental disorders.

ACADEMIC CONTEXT FOR THE TEACHING NURSING HOME

Theoretically, nowhere does the definition of nursing practice ring more true than in long-term care. The definition of nurses as persons who provide "service to the individual that helps him or her to attain or maintain a healthy state of mind or body; or, where a return to health is not possible, the relief of pain and discomfort,"[9] precisely fits the health care needs of the aged in nursing homes. Yet prior to the Teaching Nursing Home Program, it was not certain that nursing was willing to invest in nursing homes.

Health care professionals have viewed chronic illnesses afflicting nursing home patients as less solvable and less glamorous than acute care problems. Symptoms associated with chronic illnesses require intense personal care, i.e., management of incontinence, feeding, bathing, and ambulation. While physicians may be frustrated with the futility of chronic care problems, claiming that they are neither diagnostically challenging nor readily amenable to medical treatment, nurses express strong interest in such problems, and in fact have demonstrated greater success in their management than have physicians.[10]

During the 1980s schools of nursing began to allocate additional resources, such as faculty positions and clinical teaching time, to geriatrics. Mindful of professional nursing organizations' projecting a three- to fourfold increase in full-time professional nurses needed in nursing homes and encouraged by Division of Nursing (USPHS), Health and Human Services, National Institute for Mental Health and Veterans Administration funding, schools have developed and expanded masters level preparation and integration of gerontological nursing into undergraduate curricula. In 1985, there were over 50 programs preparing GNPs and gerontological clinicians and 5 preparing geropsychiatric nurses. There are over 750 practicing GNPs and over 3,000 ANA Certified Gerontological Nurses.

While these advances are indeed encouraging, we should not be misled into believing that they imply a major shift in nursing education. Most schools of nursing continue to concentrate on preparing nurses for acute care, and existing geriatric initiatives are highly vulnerable to outside pressures, such as the recently publicized nurse shortage crisis.[11]

The RWFJ TNHP Demonstration

Beginning in 1982, 11 schools of nursing and 12 nursing homes participated in this national program. The essential elements of a TNH as defined in this demonstration are:

a shared mission statement including nursing care, education (all levels), and research,

faculty appointment with clinical responsibility at the home, including teaching and research, opportunities for graduate education in nursing,

comprehension of, and commitment to interdisciplinary care of nursing home residents, and

fiscal acknowledgment of the tripartite mission of the affiliation.

While the goals of teaching and research are familiar to schools of nursing, the TNHP strategy for accomplishing these goals, i.e., the explicit requirement that nursing faculty engage in clinical practice in nursing homes, was a departure from customary relationships established between schools of nursing and clinical agencies. A few nursing (and medical) schools in the past have had contracts authorizing responsibility for clinical care of patients in Veterans Administration, city, and teaching hospitals. The TNHP, however, represented a relatively new attempt at developing such relationships with long-term care institutions.

Though the TNHP concept will ultimately be evaluated on its historic merits as a social strategy, the University of Colorado Health Science Center is conducting a national evaluation of its specific outcomes which will soon be available (see Chapter 11). In the meantime, we should ask ourselves whether encouraging the involvement of nursing schools in the care of nursing home patients proved to be an intrinsically valued idea. At least two markers are available to assess the accuracy of the original assumptions: commitment of school of nursing and nursing home resources to quality care for nursing home patients, and joint school of nursing and nursing home plans for program continuation after RWJF funding ceases. We should explore the context in which The Robert Wood Johnson Foundation Teaching Nursing Home idea was tested and examine these two markers for assessing success.

Assessing the Effect of the Demonstration

Over 90 of the more than 120 schools of nursing that were eligible to apply for RWJF-TNHP funding submitted letters of intent. Fifty-three schools and nursing homes submitted applications in response to the request for proposal. The concept of close clinical, teaching, and research linkages, therefore, was a compelling idea for a large number of schools of nursing who appeared to find no difficulty in locating potential nursing home partners.

The schools of nursing and nursing homes participating in the TNHP represented diverse institutions with varying missions and goals. They were almost equally representative of public and private universities.

Most selected sites had ongoing gerontological initiatives: three had graduate programs with gerontological majors, three sites had either an adult or geriatric nurse practitioner program, and two had some student rotations in nursing homes. Two schools had administrative responsibility for nursing services in affiliated teaching hospitals, and one also administered an affiliated skilled rehabilitation facility. In five sites, the nursing school organizational structure encouraged nursing faculty to engage in clinical practice.

The 12 participating nursing homes included two county homes, one investor-owned, one Veterans Administration, and eight voluntary homes. Four of the voluntary homes were under Roman Catholic auspices, two Methodist, one Jewish affiliated, and one nondemoninational. The Teaching Nursing Homes represented a total capacity of over 2000± beds, and ranged in size from 127 to over 500 beds. Prior to the affiliation, five homes had close corporate relationships with acute care facilities and two were part of a continuum of care including independent living units, and/or had linkages with a home health agency. While all homes had student rotations prior to the TNHP, only two had rotations from the partner university. Two had jointly funded home/university nursing positions. All but one of the original school of nursing/nursing home affiliations completed the 1982–1987 funding period. One school of nursing negotiated a new affiliation after the original affiliation dissolved in the first year.

Committing Resources

The TNHP's intrinsic value lies in the fit between program goals to provide quality care to nursing home patients, and the ability and interest of schools of nursing to respond to this need. The program proved an excellent opportunity to blend nursing home knowledge of service deficits with school of nursing and nursing home's mutual resolution to remedy these deficits. Demonstrating this commitment to better care in 1985–86, participating schools and homes supplemented TNHP funding by jointly supporting 12 FTE personnel. In addition, schools contributed approximately one-half of FTE faculty to supervise students, provide care, and conduct research in Teaching Nursing Homes in 1986–87.

Teaching Nursing Homes introduced a wide range of organizational changes aimed at improving patient care. In over half the homes, nursing services were changed from hierarchal designs to flattened, decentralized systems. Many decisions made by directors of nursing were shifted to the unit level under the supervision of head nurses who assumed 24-hour responsibility for patient care. Several homes introduced a primary care model of patient assignment whereby aides and LPNs consistently cared for one group of patients. These changes were instrumental in assuring prompt clinical decision making and in providing patients, families, and staff with an identifiable person responsible for problem resolution (see Chapter 3).

Decentralization became possible with the presence of advanced nurse clinician/faculty who were knowledgeable and experienced in geriatric care. All sites introduced geriatric nurse specialists while five sites employed the skills of gero-psychiatric nurse specialists. These clinicians, many of whom were unit based and available for consultation, assisted staff in identifying, resolving, and referring patient care problems, and significantly augmented the home's capability of caring for patients with severe illnesses.

Clinician/faculty were instrumental in assisting homes develop new clinical programs. Three sites introduced specialized units or programs for patients with dementia; three added new units for "super skilled" or highly acute patients; seven introduced or expanded home care programs, and one home initiated a respite care unit. New quality assurance programs to monitor falls, psychotropic medication use, dehydration, catheter use, etc., resulted in new facility policies, protocols and funded research studies. Ethics committees introduced in four sites resulted in explicit resuscitation policies and assured implementation of patients' wishes regarding treatment decisions and advanced directives.

All TNHPs undertook extensive inservice and continuing education programs. Learning new physical examination skills and gaining fluency in administering standardized functional and mental status examinations was a high priority. Precise knowledge of patients' physical and mental conditions is a prerequisite to accurate clinical diagnosis, appropriate nursing management, and timely referral. Five TNHPs offered continuing education (CE) courses to prepare nursing home, hospital, and home care nurses to take the ANA certification examination as Gerontological Nurse Clinicians. Over three hundred nurses completed these courses, which were usually oversubscribed. Nurse aide training also was a high TNHP priority. Six sites developed extensive nurse aide training programs, including the development of manuals which are also used in continuing education nurse aide training courses. Inservice activities included didactic classes, hands-on supervision and return demonstrations, and preparation of audio visual materials for repeated use within and outside the home. Moreover, an average of twenty-five nursing home staff per site enrolled in for-credit courses beyond their present preparation. Lastly, over three-quarters of the sites initiated patient, staff, and/or family groups. These groups, often coled by faculty and staff and/or students, served a variety of functions: reorientation and remotivation; diminishing aggressive, combative, or wandering behavior; improving functional status; dispute resolution; resolving ethical dilemmas; and encouraging family/patient involvement.

Funded research in TNHP sites represented a truly collaborative effort between the school of nursing and the nursing home. Obtaining access to patients, to staff, and to nursing home records required active nursing home collaboration. In several instances, nursing home and school of nursing personnel jointly submitted proposals. Four sites collaborated on a research proposal funded by the Division of Nursing, Health and Human Services to examine the use of a biolog unit to describe accurately the prevalence of incontinence in cognitively impaired nursing home patients.[12] This compilation suggests that, at least in these affiliations, both partners sought and found ways to commit needed resources to carry on the work of the affiliation.

Plans for Continuation

All but two of the eleven demonstration projects submitted plans for program continuation. Where affiliations are ongoing between original partners, all but one have jointly funded faculty/clinician positions. These individuals have oversight or direct responsibility for clinical care and coordination of the homes' educational and/or research programs.[13] (Funding support ranges from .05 to .1 FTE personnel.)

The willingness of homes to commit resources to project continuation in the face of severe cost and constraint is particularly impressive. Some voluntary homes have secured endowment funding for project continuation; one TNHP formed an institute to coordinate existing and new school of nursing and nursing home initiatives. A County Board of Overseers committed funding for a .5 FTE faculty/clinician position, and in one state, TNH activities will be partially sustained by a higher reimbursement for documented care by nurse clinicians. Many participating sites built on the TNHP experience competed successfully for funding of additional demonstration projects. For example, one site obtained a state contract to become a regional center for nurse aide training; another was funded to become a tri-state Geriatric Education Center (GEC).

Similarly, despite declining student enrollment and overall faculty attrition, participating schools have also made strong commitments to continue TNH activities. A major factor in the schools' continued support of gerontology faculty is their proven ability to secure outside research funding. In 1985–86, TNHP supported faculty generated almost two million dollars in additional research and program support, a sixfold increase from 1983–84 funding levels.

Two schools plan to continue existing relationships while adding new nursing home affiliates, one with a veterans administration nursing home adjacent to the university campus, and the other to manage a new 27-bed Alzheimer's unit. When one original school was unable to commit to continued affiliation, the nursing home involved allocated one FTE faculty/geriatric nurse practitioner position and now is negotiating affiliation with a new school of nursing.

Two schools terminated existing contracts with for-profit owned or managed homes. Among the reasons cited for these failed affiliations were frustration with cost constraints and frequent administrative changes. Both schools have negotiated new affiliations with not-for-profit homes. Thus, in locations familiar with a Teaching Nursing Home, the concept appears to be sufficiently enticing to encourage other nursing homes to enter into similar relationships.

CONTEXT FOR THE FUTURE

The future context for the Teaching Nursing Home is full of questions and possibly, full of promise. It seems clear, though, that the health professions are beginning to respond to the demand for nurses, doctors, social workers, and others who are prepared to work with the elderly. But, we suffer from a paucity of knowledge about aging in every sense—physiologic aging, social aging, pathophysiologic aging, and emotional aging. This ignorance makes us vulnerable and easily discouraged from instituting policies that help the elderly. After all, we may say, if there is nothing to do to help the problems of the elderly, why should we expend scarce resources on them? One of the vital functions of Teaching Nursing Homes will be to keep the problems of the aged before the eyes of the public in a way that will empower Americans to deal with the idea of being an aging society.

Another question related to value is the problem of missing financial incentives. Why should any university or, for that matter, any nursing home, get into the costly and difficult business of education and research in long-term care? Isn't the problem of care difficult enough? Isn't the problem of education sufficient? The answer, of course, is that universities and nursing homes will not embark on a Teaching Nursing Home partnership unless decisionmakers in those spheres of activity see society's support for the concept. The Teaching Nursing Home idea, which responds so well to the worries all parties have about care of the aged, may be so powerful a concept that the kind of social support needed will, indeed, be forthcoming. Teaching Nursing Homes will need the kind of subsidies that teaching hospitals get. Research money must be available to them. They will need access to some of the money earmarked for gerontological education. If they are valued, teaching nursing homes can become exemplary centers for long-term care, and this experiment in social change will continue.

REFERENCES

1. Brody E. Parent care as a normative family stress. *The Gerontologist,* 1985; 25:94–98.
2. Weissart W. Some reasons why it is so difficult to make community-based care cost-effective. *Health Services Research* 1985; 20:423–433.
3. U.S. Senate Special Committee on Aging. *Aging in America: Trends and Projections.* Washington DC: January, 1988.
4. Institute of Medicine. *Improving the quality of care in nursing homes.* Washington DC: National Academy Press, 1986.
5. Strahan G. Nursing Home Characteristics; Preliminary data from the 1985 National Nursing Home Survey, Hyattsville MD: National Center for Health Statistics, (Advanced Data Number 131), March 27, 1987.
6. Health Care Financing Administration. National health expenditures, 1986–2000. *Health Care Financing Review* 1987; 8:1–36.
7. Richardson, H, & Kovner, T. Swing beds: Current experience and future directions. *Health Affairs,* Fall 1987; 6 (3)p. 61–74.
8. Institute of Medicine, op.cit.
9. Henderson V. *The Nature of Nursing.* New York: MacMillan Co. 1961, p. 15.
10. Runyan J W. The Memphis chronic disease program, comparisons in outcome, the nurse's expanded role. *JAMA* 1975; 236:264–267.
11. Aiken, L H, Mullinex C F. The nurse shortage: myth or reality? *New England Journal of Medicine,* 1987; 317:641–646.
12. Colling J, Ouslander J, Hadley B J, Campbell E, Eisch J. *Patterned urge–response toileting for urinary incontinence.* Washington DC: NIH-NCNR Grant #NR01554-02.
13. Colling J, Gamroth L: Teaching Nursing Home Program leads to creation of Institute for Long Term Care Practice at Benedictine Center. *Provider News (Teaching Nursing Home Supplement),* Washington DC; American Association of Homes for the Aging, April 15, 1988.

2

Patient's Needs, Societal Resources, and Nursing Strategies

William L. Kissick and Karen K. Knibbe

DEFINITION OF NEED

"Grow old with me the best is yet to be." These immortal words written by Robert Browning to his wife Elizabeth Barrett Browning, articulate one vision of the aging process. One wonders what Robert Browning might have written had he been a biomedical scientist, medical gerontologist, or gerontological nurse practitioner. He would likely have perceived needs for economic security, social support, health care, and nursing home services. But what of those needs? How are they to be measured? And how are they to be met? What resources are available? What are the resultant nursing strategies?

Although we tend to think of nursing home needs collectively, they are in the final analysis, singular. We may aggregate individual patient's needs but still fail to appreciate collective need. Moreover, societies in attempting to allocate resources to meet population health care requirements often fail to meet the needs of individual patients.

In the health professions, as with many other human services, we tend to confuse the individual with the statistical average. While there are individuals, and individuals may be aggregated as population groups, there are still no average individuals. Each is a distinct person. One can think of an individual person and a statistical person but not an average person.

We acknowledge the dilemma of trying to express individual patient needs in terms of collective data. Further, we stipulate that even though health care strategies which allocate societal resources to meet patients' needs are often founded on statistics, they must have their ultimate effect on the individual patient. A strategy developed to be appropriate for the statistical person is not always applicable to each of the individuals constituting the statistic.

Let us therefore, begin with a case presentation of an individual and her needs. We shall then describe several perceptions by others of that individual. As we search for ways to meet the needs of the singular person we shall look to societal resources and societal priorities. Finally, we pose a question for nursing strategy. How can nursing respond to both statistical needs and those of the individual patient . . . the one who provoked our search in the first place?

CASE PRESENTATION

Patient History

Mrs. S., an 83-year-old woman, has been widowed for 20 years. Her husband, who died at age 65, was a self-employed carpenter all his working life. Mrs. S. was never employed and left school in the sixth grade. She was a homemaker and mother of two; a son, now 65 years old and living out of state with his own family, and a daughter, now 63 years old and living with her own family two miles from the three-story home Mr. and Mrs. S. had owned and lived in their entire married life. Her only source of income is a monthly Social Security check of $353.

One and a half years ago, when she was no longer capable of living alone, Mrs. S. sold her home and moved in with her daughter's family. Even though, for the most part, she enjoyed good health, she was disabled by bilateral cataracts, severe arthritis of her hands, knees, and feet, decreased hearing, and a slight loss of memory. She could no longer prepare her own meals, and her diet-controlled, noninsulin dependent diabetes worsened. She could not use the telephone, leave her home without assistance, maintain her housekeeping chores, or remember when or what medications she needed to take.

While living with her daughter, Mrs. S. was cheerful. Her soft speech was rambling, chattering, albeit coherent. In spite of severe arthritis of her hands, she was able to feed herself. Her appetite was good and her diabetes came under control. She was able to use a walker and could ambulate moderate distances otherwise unaided. She went to the bathroom alone and was able to get into bed by herself. She could not button, zip, or close hooks when dressing, nor could she wash her back or legs while bathing. She also needed help with taking her medications (one-half tablet of Digoxin every day, one tablet of Lasix each morning, and one caplet of Ibuprofen twice a day) because of her forgetfulness as well as difficulty in opening medication bottles. That was all the help she required from anyone—before the fall!

Mrs. S. required a three-week hospitalization for a surgical pinning of her fractured left femur. Upon admission to the hospital, she was confused as to time, place, and events, however, she retained awareness of her own and her family's identity and her date of birth. During the hospitalization, her mental status declined; she no longer recognized her family. She became incontinent of bowel and bladder. With discharge planning, nursing home placement became a consideration. Much deliberation and consultation ensued with physicians, nurses, and the hospital social worker and finally the family decided to place Mrs. S. in a nursing home until her condition improved. At discharge, Mrs. S. remained incontinent and confused about her environment, time, and identity of others, but still capable of feeding herself.

During the third week in the nursing home, the staff noted increased confusion in Mrs. S. She no longer remembered how to use the walker without repeated directions and encouragement, could not state her name and birth date, and forgot how to use a fork and spoon. Her pleasant chatter lost its coherency and turned into moans and groans. In addition to forgetting how to eat, Mrs. S. began to have difficulty chewing and seemed to lose her appetite. While she continued to be incontinent, her output decreased and her urine became very concentrated and foul. Her drowsy day time periods increased and she became harder to arouse from sleep.

Her physical status changed also, though less drastically. Her blood pressure fluctuated slightly from 120/60 to 108/50 while her temperature increased from her normal 97.5 to 98.8 degrees. Her breathing while resting became shallow and the rate increased from her normal 18 to 30 breaths per minute. Her resting heart rate increased from 78 to 88 beats per minute and on moderate activity it increased even more. Both feet and ankles showed increased moderate swelling but remained warm to the touch. Mrs. S.'s state of health declined rapidly.

Family Perspective

My mother, Mrs. S., has deteriorated so drastically in the past several weeks. It is difficult to imagine her as ever being an independent woman, let alone being able to return to her state of semi-dependence before the fall. My family and I are sad to see her in this condition. Before her illness she was a strong, pleasant, gracious, and popular woman. If only she didn't have to suffer her remaining life in a nursing home, but there was no way we could have afforded her nursing care in our home. I gave up my job as a cook in the local grade school so I could be with her and help her. Now my family has no extra income. I know too, that at my age (63), I would not have been able to care for her myself because of my arthritis. It was difficult to do this to my mother . . . putting her in a nursing home . . . but under the circumstances, it was our only choice.

We are pleased with the care she is receiving in the nursing home. We are kept informed of her changing condition and we always have someone to talk with if we have questions. The nurse practitioner and doctor have been available to us and we feel as though the entire staff is working together to help my mother.

Now that she is on Medicaid, we are so relieved! Without it, we would never be able to afford this good care unless we sold our home. My mother has already spent her life savings just to receive the care she is getting. She always said she would rather die than be on welfare, but if she had a choice now, I know she would give in and accept it. And she is actually contributing to the cost of her care. Her Social Security check of $353 per month goes toward paying the bill.

Physician Impression

I came to know Mrs. S. in the hospital when I was asked by her surgeon to evaluate her for surgery. I saw her periodically throughout her hospitalization to regulate her medications and her medical care. Now I continue my involvement with her in the teaching nursing home.

I have my own private practice as well as a teaching appointment in the medical school that is associated with the hospital and the teaching nursing home. My routine visits to the nursing home are limited to two afternoons per week at the most and each visit to her is reimbursed by third-party payment. I am available for phone consultation with the nurse practitioner.

Mrs. S. is an elderly woman who is dealing with a progressive decline of systems functions . . . cardiac, respiratory, urinary . . . along with mental and physical functions. My role in her care is to ascertain a need for medical management of these functions. In the elderly, symptoms are vague, and many times unspecific. The whole picture of the patient is necessary before treatment can be prescribed.

The nurse practitioner and I have collaborated on management protocols that enable the nurse practitioner to change the medical management when needed based on findings of the patient assessment. When changes in the patient's condition necessitates actions not covered by the protocol, I change the medical plan. Since I see the patient less frequently than the nurse practitioner, I depend on the telephone consultations with the nurse to base my medical judgments.

Sharing of information is necessary among all the disciplines involved in the care of Mrs. S. The nurse practitioner coordinates the communication and when necessary, calls a team conference which I attend as a team member.

If rehospitalization is indicated, I continue my involvement with Mrs. S. on a daily basis as her primary care physician. Then it is my turn to keep the nurse practitioner informed of Mrs. S.'s status while in the hospital. Upon return to the nursing home, the nurse practitioner takes over the primary management of Mrs. S. and informs me of changes if they occur when I am not present.

Nursing Strategy

I am a master's prepared nurse practitioner and am employed full time in this teaching nursing home. I have been following Mrs. S. since her admission three weeks ago. Her decline in overall condition requires me to become more involved in her daily care since her whole being is compromised by her physical status.

My goal in caring for Mrs. S. is to assist her to maintain wholeness by adapting to changes in her state of health and in her environment. My approach to her care is based on three separate but related elements that aid me in planning my nursing actions: 1) a conceptual model of nursing care based on an ongoing assessment of the needs of Mrs. S. and her family; 2) a determination of the functional and mental status of Mrs. S.; and 3) a determination of the cause and extent of physical and biological changes associated with Mrs. S.'s declining state of health.

My role as a nurse practitioner in the teaching nursing home is of the utmost importance in the care of Mrs. S. for several reasons. First, by basing my nursing actions on extensive daily functional, mental, and physical assessments, I practice advanced nursing. Along with ordering nursing measures to maintain her integrity, provide reorientation and the like, I will order the necessary laboratory work, alter her medications, and perhaps start a broad spectrum of antibiotics. I might order a chest x-ray and an electrocardiogram to determine whether she requires medical intervention. I keep her physician informed of all that I have found and my plan of action.

Second, I am in the nursing home every day and can immediately respond to reported changes in her condition. Because my services are salaried, each involvement and assessment requires no consultation fee.

Third, I teach the nursing home staff how to provide the best care possible to each individual based on the latest nursing and medical research findings. I am a role model for the staff and a formal instructor on nursing and patient care issues.

Fourth, I coordinate the care Mrs. S. receives by collaborating with the professional nursing staff and nursing assistants, physicians, the physical therapist, speech therapist, and the social worker. My coordinating role assures mutual goal planning across all the disciplines through adequate and accurate communication. Mrs. S.'s family is an integral part of the team and their involvement is always included in planning for her care.

In sum, my role as nurse practitioner in the teaching nursing home is a vital one to assure adequate and appropriate delivery of nursing and medical care in a nonfragmented, cost-effective manner. Both Mrs. S. and her family are the recipients of the multidisciplinary approach to care based on their individual needs. In this way, quality of care and ultimately quality of life can be best achieved.

Administrator's View

I am trying to run a quality nursing home with the least cost and the greatest amount of reimbursement (private pay or third-party) as possible. To provide quality care, I need well-prepared nurses, good nursing assistants, and physicians knowledgeable in the care of the elderly. I also need adequate equipment, good referral sources, and a positive image in the community to maintain our services. The hardest part is to remain financially solvent since most of our reimbursement for care is by Medicaid which reimburses at a much lower per diem rate than Medicare or private pay. Professional nurses provide quality care but they are scarce and expensive. The least expensive and most available worker is the untrained nursing assistant but then quality care is sacrificed, our positive image in the community is threatened, and a "Catch-22" situation results.

We have recently hired a nurse practitioner who has added to our efficiency, quality, and image, but is expensive because of salary, benefits, and indirect costs. Because part of her role includes education and training of our staff, the indirect costs of nonproductive educational time have risen. Also, the number of nursing hours per patient by the nurse practitioner and the rest of the staff is many times skewed in the direction of spending more time on patients who generate less income.

For example, Mrs. S. has been here for three weeks. Despite her illness, she does not qualify for skilled nursing care and therefore, is not eligible for Medicare reimbursement. She has exhausted her private assets and is now on Medicaid. Because of her acuity, the nurse practitioner has spent increasing time with her family, and the staff caring for her. While I am sure the best care for Mrs. S. is being provided under these circumstances, I also am sure that our nursing home is losing money.

In the short term, nurse practitioner care for Mrs. S. is a losing deal financially, but a winning deal in quality of care. In the long-term, I hope that with improved services, a better educated staff, and perhaps expanded services of the nursing staff into the community that can generate income, we'll have a winning deal financially and in quality.

Taxpayer's Concern

I've known Mrs. S. and her family since I moved to this area ten years ago. I'm sorry that this has happened to her and her family. But the basic issues come down to just a few questions.

How long will the costs for health care remain so high? Everything I read tells me there is no end in sight. As our society continues to get older, more and more dollars will go to take care of people just like Mrs. S. who spend a long time in the hospital . . . costing the taxpayers huge amounts of dollars . . . and [the people will] not be able to return to a productive life. In fact, now she needs more care, more dollars, and she will probably die without knowing all society has done for her.

What about my children? With few tax dollars going to their education and the increase in the cost of living, how will I be able to pay for all they need? Is it fair to take away from the young who have a productive future and give it to the old who have none?

What would I want if Mrs. S. were my mother whose health is failing too? Even though my mother is 69 years old and living in her own home, I can see the day drawing nearer that she will need help. What then? Will there be enough dollars for health care left for her? Will others feel about her the way I feel about Mrs. S.?

What will happen when my wife and I need the care Mrs. S. is now receiving? Will there be enough money to pay for us when we need help? What will happen to us if our children can't or won't take care of us?

I don't have the answers. It seems as though we could come up with more money, more answers, better care. I am frustrated with the system, the government, and Mrs. S., although I have sympathy for her and her family at the same time. What a dilemma? Who has a right to our dwindling societal economic resources. Who decides?

NEEDS AND REQUIREMENTS FOR HEALTH CARE

Any statement of need for health services is, to a certain degree, arbitrary. Therefore, the boundaries of needs must be established. Few would disagree that a person suffering from acute appendicitis is in need of a surgeon. Likewise, a patient with diabetic acidosis is in need of an array of health services to save his life. Epidemiology seeks to determine incidence and prevalence of disease as a measure of need. But in most areas need is determined by a highly judgmental process. How many times does a patient with well-controlled diabetes or hypertension need to seek professional care? How many times ought an infant, during the first year of life, see a pediatrician or pediatrician nurse practitioner? If one final definitive answer could be cited to each of these questions, a specified need for health services could be determined.

Economists and health specialists agree that forecasts based on a finite need for future health services are unrealistic. Instead they suggest forecasting in terms of demand for health services in the classic economic sense of supply and demand. For the most part, demand is the economic expression of need, but some suggest demand may be beyond actual need. Illustrative of this point of view is the affluent hypochondriac who may be expressing a demand for health services that is in excess of actual needs. Others feel that anxiety expressed by a patient for a physician's services is a valid need and not an inappropriate demand.

The purchasing power of the aged for health services has increased with the establishment of the Medicare program in 1965; it is estimated that expenditures will exceed $100 billion per day by the next decade. Many take the position that this increased purchasing power, whatever the amount, will allow the aged to translate needs into demand, while others state that this will allow the aged to generate demand for health services in excess of actual need.

In many respects the requirements for health services can be virtually insatiable, depending on a society's level of expectation and the resources it wishes to allocate. At any rate, it would appear that any characterization of the dimension, quantitative and qualitative, of requirements for health services is arbitrarily defined. In the case history above we had six perceptions of need and demand—the patient, the family, the physician, the nurse practitioner, the nursing home administrator, and the taxpayer. All are valid. How do we synthesize or choose? Who shall decide?

Health Status and Health Services Utilization

Preliminary data demonstrates that about 19% of 65 plus persons have some degree of limitation (mild to severe): 16% are males and 21% are females.[1] More than 80% of persons 65 and over have at least one chronic condition, and multiple conditions are commonplace in the elderly. The leading chronic conditions causing limitation of activity for the elderly in 1982 were arthritis and hypertensive disease, hearing impairments, and heart conditions. Osteoporisis is much more common among older women than in men while coronary heart disease is much more common among the older men. Heart disease leads all other conditions in the indicators of health care utilization.[2] Estimates of the prevalence of incontinence in the elderly range from 5–20% among persons living in the community.[3] While its prevalence is unknown, many geriatric psychiatrists believe that about 10% of the population over 65 suffer from depression.[4]

In 1977, Brody reported that 32% of the elderly had no limitations on their activities. Seven percent have some limitation but not on their major activity, while 30% do. Approximately 15% are unable to carry out their major activity.[5] Preliminary data from the 1982 National Long-Term Care Survey (NLTCS) demonstrated that among the non-institutionalized disabled population 19% of the 65 plus persons have one degree of limitation (mild to severe): 16% of males and 21% of females. Four percent of the elderly population is severely disabled: 3% of males and 4% of females. Although more than half of the 85 plus generation are not disabled, cross-sectional data demonstrates that the chance of becoming at lease mildly disabled increases for the oldest age groups.[6]

More than 33% of all elderly disabled members living in the community are cared for by a wife, while only 10% of elderly disabled women are cared for by a husband. Children of aging parents provide care to about 25% of elderly males in this category and to slightly over 33% of elderly women. About 5% of the elderly population are in nursing homes at any given time. Of this group, approximately 50% are severely disabled with Alzheimer's or a related disease causing mental impairment.[7]

The average length of stay in a hospital for persons age 65 to 74 was about 9 days in 1983 compared with about 11 days for the 85 year and over group.[8] Eleven percent of visits to physicians in 1980 were by people over the age 65.[9] Seventy-five percent of the elderly had been prescribed at least one prescription drug in 1977.[10]

Home health care is becoming an increasingly important option of care for the elderly. Among the aged Medicare beneficiaries in 1983 (those over the age of 65), the number of persons per 1,000 enrollees receiving home health agency services was higher for the increasingly older age groups. The user rate for persons 85 years of age or over was eight times higher than the rate for persons aged 65–66. The number of persons per 1,000 enrollees receiving home health services was more than 50% higher for the aged than the non-aged disabled, but the average number of visits per user was much higher for the disabled than for the aged.[11]

Total Medicare reimbursement for home health care increased almost twelvefold from $0.14 billion in 1974 to $1.67 billion in 1984, an average annual compounded growth rate of 28% and nearly 3.0% of the total Medicare expenditures.[12] On the other hand, Medicaid expenditures for home health care in 1983 was approximately $597 million, slightly less than 1.9% of the total Medicaid expenditures and with an annual compounded growth rate of 21.6% between 1980–1983.[13]

Collectively, Medicare and Medicaid expenditures are much greater for institutional care than for non-institutional long-term care. In 1982, Medicare and Medicaid spent only $1.7 billion for home health care compared to the $27 billion spent collectively on nursing home care. Of that $27 billion, Medicaid is the principal source of public payments (49% of the total), with Medicare paying 2%, private insurance paying 1%, and "out-of-pocket" private spending comprising all the rest.[14] It is notable that the elderly poor represent 15–17% of all Medicaid recipients, but account for 40% of program payments.[15]

As noted above, the amount of private expenditures for nursing home care is significant, however, out-of-pocket spending by the elderly for home health care is also rising. Estimates from industry in 1979 of private insurance and out-of-pocket expenditures for home health care were $1.7 billion compared to $2.3 billion in 1981, a rapid increase.[16] Out-of-pocket expenses for the elderly are not equal to those prior to the enactment of Medicare and Medicaid.[17]

Economic Security of the Elderly

The myth that the elderly are generally poorer than the nonelderly, prevalent even a decade ago, recently has been superseded by the myth that they are now better off than the nonelderly. With increased benefits from Cost of Living Adjustments (COLA) to Social Security, a greater portion of new retirees receiving pension funds, and some with private assets, one could question why, if the elderly are really as well off as they seem, do they have a preferential claim on societal dollars to pay for health care costs.

To respond to these questions, let us look at the elderly population by using Mrs. S. (our case study) as a statistical person.

> Mrs. S. is 83 years old, a widow of a self-employed capenter (who died at the age of 65 in 1967), after being eligible to contribute to the Social Security fund since the early 1950s. Mrs. S. was never employed and therefore did not accrue taxable wages to develop her own fund. Her only income is a monthly Social Security check of $353 based on survivor's benefits. She had

no income from assets until after the sale of her house. However, the balance of that asset, according to her daughter, was spent during the first three weeks of her nursing home stay.

Mrs. S. is one of the 91% of all persons over the age of 65 to receive benefits from Social Security and one of the 14% to depend totally on the benefits as the only source of income. Sixty-two percent of the elderly depend on Social Security for at least half of their income and 24% of the elderly depend on it for 90% of their income.[18] Also, Mrs. S. is one of the 42% of women aged 65 years and older who receive benefits based solely on their husband's earning records.[19]

Mrs. S.'s monthly income was far below the 1984 average monthly benefits for widows and widowers in her same age group of 75 to 84. Mrs. S. was receiving $353 while the average in her cohort was $437. Of those aged 85 years and older, the average monthly income was $400.[20] Mrs. S. was maintaining her existence with a poverty level income, which in 1984 was $4,979 per year.[21]

Being an elderly woman living alone places one at a great risk for a poverty situation. According to the United States Bureau of the Census (1980), the poverty rate among elderly women is 19%, the highest for any age group in the United States. Of the total number of elderly poor, 72% are women.[22] Of these elderly poor women, 90% are those who never married, or who are widowed, separated, or divorced. To compare the sexes, in 1984 67% of women age 75 years and older were widowed while 67% of the men in this age group were still married. And in 1983 65% of men age 78 and older lived with their wives while only 21% of women over age 75 lived with their husbands.[23]

How does the income of the old-elderly compare with that of the new retirees since 1980? To begin with, pensions, earnings, and income from assets along with Social Security benefits are the major sources of income for the largest number of recently retired workers. When pensions (public and private) and tax deferred savings (Keogh and IRAs) are considered, approximately 50% of the men, 40% of the unmarried men and women, and almost 25% of the married women receive such income. Of the newly retired workers, nearly 80% receive asset income from interest, dividends, rental property, roomers or boarders, estates, trusts, or royalties, and repayment on personal loans. Less than 2% of the newly retired workers who received the first of the Social Security benefits reported in 1982 that they were receiving cash assistance— either Supplemental Security Income or state and local welfare payments—to bring people above the poverty line.[24]

In comparing Mrs. S. and her cohort to the newly retired elderly, one can readily see that more women are in the younger group than before and they continue to earn fewer dollars than their male counterparts. When breaking up the incomes into quarters for easier comparison, women comprise 60% of those men and women in the lowest quartile, and 4% of those in the highest. The median amount of income from all sources to the newly retired workers was $18,100 for men and their wives, $17,700 for married women and their husbands, $9,300 for unmarried men, and $9,100 for unmarried women.[25]

To conclude, the belief that the elderly are well off and should be able to pay for their own health care is also a myth. It can be best summed by J. H. Schultz (1985) who wrote in *The Economics of Aging:*[26]

> From a statistical point of view, the elderly in this country are beginning to look a lot like the rest of the population; some very rich, lots with adequate income, lots more with very modest incomes (often near poverty), and a *significant minority still* destitute.

SOCIETAL RESOURCES

The resources of any society regardless of its geographic location, racial or ethnic composition, history, traditions, and political structures are basically people, knowledge, and wealth. In the United States these terms are translated into labor force, state of the art, and capital. Each of these resources has relatively finite limits.

A population is the source of the providers as well as the patients. The age and sex profile of a society is fundamental to its destiny. In the age of high tech and complex communication, educational status is critical. Some would argue that the state of the art or the knowledge base is infinite. In a sense, we can never learn everything. Admittedly, the advance of biomedical sciences had been as dramatic as other technoscientific events in our society such as lasers, computers, satellites, and robots. These marvels notwithstanding, the boundaries of ignorance are infinite. Our capital (our dollars, our productivity, our entrepreneurial initiative and achievement) is the measure of the means available to address problems. The most frequently cited index of societal resources is the Gross National Product (GNP), the sum total of all the goods and services produced in our economy.

All of us, whether nurse, physician, or health care administrator has heard the familiar conviction, "No matter what it costs, we want the best for our (father, mother, spouse, or child.)" Although often consciously expressed by individuals in time of acute crisis or medical emergency, the aspiration can be applied throughout the spectrum of health care. In contrast, society makes choices consciously and unconsciously. There are societal priorities. The painful truth is that a dollar spent on health care cannot be spent on education or, for that matter, food, housing, clothing, transportation, recreation, or conservation. And so, we come to the real conflict between societal priorities and patient needs.

"No cost is too great to save a human life" is the medical perspective which stands in conflict with the societal perspective, "Resources by definition are limited and choices must be made." No society, now matter how wealthy, can afford to provide all of the health and medical care its population is capable of consuming or, for that matter, requires. It is in this context that the Teaching Nursing Home attempts to cope with the dilemma of societal resources and patient needs through a nursing strategy.

Health Personnel

In any human service endeavor such as health care, personnel or the labor force is the most critical basic resource. When one hears the terms health personnel or health manpower, one usually thinks of physicians, nurses, and dentists. Indeed there are 2.1 million nurses (1986 total of RNs and LPNs), outnumbering 560,000 physicians almost 4:1. When you add 100,000 dentists, the total of these professions represents less than one-half of the health labor force of six million. The other half of the health labor force (three million individuals) constitute more than three dozen occupational categories, e.g., physical therapy, podiatry, optometry, and pharmacy and one million workers in the areas of secretarial, communications, maintenance, security, and other support staff that are common to many industries. When specialization is identified there are hundreds of vocational subcategories.

Moreover, these occupational groups represent career preparations that range from on-the-job-training (OJT) following a grade school education or even less, to 12, 13, 14, and 15 years or more of higher education. In the late 1980s how do we evaluate the provision of care by a nurse practitioner (an 18th grader) and a family physician (a 24th grader at a minimum)? This is but one of the many health personnel challenges we face in allocating societal resources to meet patient's needs.

Facilities

The National Nursing Home Survey (NNHS) conducted by the National Center for Health Statistics[27] reports an estimated 19,100 nursing homes in the United States in 1985 provided more than 1,624,100 beds. This is a 22% increase in the number of nursing homes since 1973–1974 and 38% increase in the number of beds. The single most important measure of nursing home utilization is an occupancy rate, which estimates that nursing homes operated at about 92% of capacity in 1984. This is a significant increase over the 1972 rate of 85.6%. Approximately 1.3

million admissions to nursing homes occurred in 1985 compared to 1.2 million discharges due to either death or placement elsewhere.

It is important to remember that no two nursing homes are really alike. They come in all shapes, sizes, and sponsorship. There are 3,800 voluntary, nonprofit nursing homes, accounting for almost 23% of the beds and 20% of the total number of institutions. Public institutions (VA, state, county, and municipal) make up only 8.1% of the beds; they represent approximately 3% of the institutions. By far, the largest number of nursing homes are proprietary, 75%, and account for 69% of the number of beds.

Biomedical Research

The post-World War II investment in biomedical research was launched in 1946 when the National Heart Institute was authorized as a companion to the National Cancer Institute which had been established in 1937. Thus began the proliferation of institutes, the National Institutes on Aging being the most recently established, that now constitute the National Institutes of Health. The national investment over the past two decades is measured in tens of billions.

During the past four decades we have witnessed a virtual cornucopia of biomedical advances and technological innovations, for example: Tranquilizers, beta blockers, H2 inhibitors, cyclosporin, laser surgery, lithotripters, total hip arthroplasty, cardiac angiography, coronary artery by-pass grafts (CABG), organ transplantation, magnetic resonance imaging, and end stage renal dialysis. Marvelous? Yes, but remember cost-effective utilization is challenged. Moreover, what are the ultimate cost-benefit implications for the very old who have a limited life expectancy? Many Mrs. S.'s have benefited from total hip arthroplasties. How does one evaluate the potential benefits against the cost?

THE RISE OF A VAST INDUSTRY

For the years immediately following World War II and throughout the 1950s national health policy focused on the investment of public funds in the development of the basic resources—health personnel, health care facilities, and biomedical research. There was an implicit assumption that the allocation of resources would follow automatically and services would be provided. Subsequently it was recognized that all industries depend on the translation of basic resources into goods and services called the "production function" or "entrepreneurial factor." In the health care systems financing mechanisms and organizational patterns constitute delivery systems as the "production function" that orchestrates basic resources into health services.

Financing

Financing of health care since the origin of Blue Cross in 1929 has evolved into a maze of inconsistencies, exceptions, adaptations, and almost incomprehensible regulations. In most market endeavors we are accustomed to paying out-of-pocket in exchange for a service. In health care, only three of every ten dollars are paid out-of-pocket by the consumer. Three dollars come from third-party insurance and four dollars come from the government. Moreover, the portion of the total varies by product or service. For example, only 5% of hospital costs are out-of-pocket in contrast to the vast majority of prescription costs. We pay for health care by very different routes.

Now we look at the dynamics of the transactions. Rather than the two party interaction of most markets (the buyer and seller), the patient (party of the first part), consults a physician (party of the second part), who sends a bill to Blue Shield (party of the third part), who sells a contract to the employer (party of the fourth part), who provides the employee (party of the first part), fringe benefits in lieu of wages. Not surprisingly, accountability gets lost in multiple transactions.

This is the area entered by Medicare and Medicaid in 1965. For two decades hundreds of billions of dollars were poured into a nonmarket, poorly regulated, and essentially nondisciplined system. The United States Congress after almost two decades of frustration over health care cost escalation authorized Prospective Cost Based Payment with DRGs (Diagnostic Related Groups). Now by the authority vested in the Department of Health and Human Services by the United States Congress there are 467 diagnostic categories by which hospitals will be reimbursed prospectively by Medicare regardless of costs incurred to the institution.

Organization

This brings us to the organization and delivery of health services. Notwithstanding the credo of solo practice for American medicine, the Mayo, Ochsner, Cleveland, and Leahy Clinics stand out as models of corporate practice. Multihospital systems, corporate restructuring, and investor-owned corporations such as Health Corporation of America, Humana, and National Medical Enterprise are macroorganizations. Some predict that virtually all hospitals will be part of multihospital systems by the year 2000. The organizational initiatives getting the most actions are HMOs, Preferred Provider Organization, and Medical Staff/ Hospital-Joint Ventures. The corporate practice of medicine would appear to be in the midst of a transformation from the pariah of the 1950s and 1960s to the panacea of the 21st century.

NURSING STRATEGIES IN TEACHING NURSING HOMES

Nursing traditionally has recognized that while compelled to do everything possible for the individual patient, one could not do everything for all the patients for whom one is responsible during an eight-hour shift. The issue of cost–quality tradeoff, increasingly discussed by the medical profession and health care managers, has long been a reality for nurses confronted by limited time and material resources. This truism of nursing must be recognized as the first principle of the Teaching Nursing Home and a priority lesson for the broader health care enterprise in our society. "No cost is too great to save a human life, treat disease, or make a patient comfortable." "Resources by definition are limited and choices must be made." These are the respective convictions of medicine and management in health affairs. Nursing has long been the health profession that has attempted to address both forms of this dilemma.

The organizational structure of the voluntary hospital, as it grew to dominance in the post-World War II era, has been diagramed and discussed in terms of the dual authority of administration and medical staff reporting to the board of trustees. The "Iron Triangle" is illustrated below, with nursing *de jure* employed by hospital administrators but *de facto* serving physicians who write the orders, or in the era of DRGs, determine the "product line." Many a nurse has actually dominated the play by an adroit mastery of the "Doctor–Nurse Game."[28]

A vast literature, including textbooks, have been devoted to analysis of this power structure in eleemosynary health care institutions. Often nursing has been treated as an afterthought, within the domain of administration, exhibited on many organizational charts. Functionally, however, nursing has been *the* critical element in a hospital system. After all, hospitals provide mainly nursing services. The designation, "Teaching Nursing Home" connotes a reality of function and mission as well as a demand for clarity of structure.

The functional diagram for a voluntary hospital may be *de jure* as illustrated above. But with the advent of DRGs, nursing has become *de facto* the interface between the administration and the medical staff, joined by the (resonant bonds of organic chemistry) which provide the stability of interdependence to the institution and its derivative relationships.

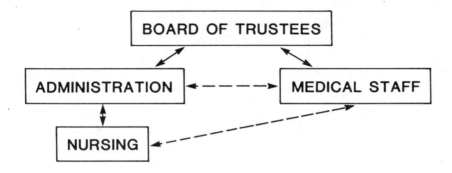

Figure 2.1 Iron triangle of hospital structure.

The organizational scheme for Teaching Nursing Homes suggests that professional nurses are evolving to a new stage by serving *quasi* medical staff functions and administrative responsibilities as well as traditional nursing services. Thus, nursing moves to the center of the "Iron Triangle" diagramed above with linkages to institutional governance, administration, and medical services to cope with cost–quality tradeoffs, the likely dominant theme for health affairs in the 21st century.

Closed Budgets

When Medicare and Medicaid were enacted in 1965, our society launched expenditures of hundreds of billions of dollars of public funds over ensuing decades to finance health services for the elderly and the medically indigent. These funds were expended in a health care economy undisciplined by the marketplace or the public sector. The resulting cost inflation occurred on an unprecedented scale. Health care expenditures in 1965 totaling approximately $80 billion accounted for 5.8% of Gross National Product. The $458 billion expended in 1986 accounted for 10.9% of Gross National Product. The Health Care Financing Administration forecasts $1.5 *trillion* representing 15% of Gross National Product in the year 2000.[29] An extrapolation of these trends would reach 100% of Gross National Product by the year 2057.

Obviously health care expenditures are on an escalator that is destined to top out. If the American health care system does not prepare itself for the inevitable plateau in expenditures the crunch is certain to be traumatic, if not devastating, to all the components. Anticipatory strategies are imperative for cost-effective health care achievements.

From Patients to Constituents

Nursing has many lessons for health care systems. Years ago a nurse, who had served as an airline stewardess prior to attending nursing school, came into the doctors office of a major teaching hospital late one night and asked to the intern to, "Look in on the passenger in the room at the end of the hall." The request was insightful and provocative. We treat passengers quite differently from patients. The term patient derives from the Latin "to suffer." The nursing model incorporates passengers while the medical model is limited to patients.

"Teaching Nursing Homes" by its title, implies institutions in which the nursing model is more critical than the medical model. As our patients become passengers, they are becoming subscribers, beneficiaries, clients, consumers, and customers. We need to think of them as constituents—with reciprocal accountability. We are accountable to them as they are dependent on us. In the Wharton School at the University of Pennsylvania the term "stakeholders" is a concept aimed at broadening the term shareholder to encompass all vested interests. Stakeholders can be those who work for an organization, customers, governments, communities, or suppliers. As we look at our individual responsibilities for patient's needs and societal priorities, one can be assured that in the 21st century we shall all be the stakeholders.

Moreover, the stakeholders—Mrs. S. and her family, the physician, the nurse, the administrator, and the taxpayer—discussed in the case history at the outset of this chapter, are all part of the effort to balance patient's needs and societal resources. Institutional reforms are imperative if we are to translate our vast resources into equity, excellence, and cost-effectiveness in health care for the elderly. Our society can tolerate no less than health care of appropriate quality for all its citizens. We can afford no more. Teaching Nursing Homes mandate nursing strategies to address the dilemma of balancing patients needs with societal resources in the 21st century.

REFERENCES

1. Manton K G, Liu K. *The future growth of the long-term care population: Projections based on the 1977 National Nursing Home Survey and the 1982 Long-Term Care Survey.* In *America in Transition: An Aging Society,* Serial No. 99-B. Washington DC: U.S. Government Printing Office, 1985.
2. U.S. Bureau of Census. Prepared by Jacob S. Siegel. *Demographic and Socioeconomic Aspects of Aging in the United States* (Series p-23, No. 138) Special Committee on Aging Report, U.S. Senate. Washington, DC: U.S. Government Printing Office; 1985:67.

3. Rowe J W. Health care of the elderly. *N Engl J Med.* 1985; 312 (13): 827–834.
4. Charaton F B. Depression and the elderly. *Psychiatric Annals,* 1985; 15(5): 313–316.
5. Brody E M. Aging. *Encyclopedia of Social Work.* Silver Spring, MD: National Association of Social Workers; 1977: 55–78.
6. Manton K G, Liu K, op cit.
7. Jette A M, Branch L G. The Framingham Disability Study: Physical disability among the aging. *Am. J. Public Health* 1981; 71(1): 1211–1216.
8. Special Committee on Aging. *America in Transition: An Aging Society* (Rep. No. 46–295, Serial No. 99–B). Washington, DC: U.S. Government Printing Office, 1985; 12–73.
9. Ibid. p. 75.
10. Ibid. p. 78.
11. Kirby W, Latta B, Hibling C. Health care financing trends: Medicare use and cost of home health agency services, 1983–84. *Health Care Financing Review,*
12. Ibid. p. 95.
13. Ibid. p. 93.
14. Doty P, Liu K, Wiener J. An overview of long-term care. *Health Care Financing Rev.* 1985; 6(3): 73–75.
15. Ibid. p. 78.
16. Upp M. Fast facts and figures about social security. *Soc. Secur. Bull.* 1986; 49(6):15.
17. Doty P., Liu K, Wiener J, op cit. p. 72.
18. Special Committee on Aging, op. cit. p. 4.
19. Upp M, op. cit. p. 8. Ibid. p. 8.
20. Ibid. p. 14.
21. Upp M. Fast Facts and Figures About Social Security. *Soc. Secur. Bull.* 1986; 49(6):11. Ibid. p. 11.
22. Upp M. Fast Facts and Figures About Social Security. *Soc. Secur. Bull.* (1986; 49 6; 6. Ibid. p. 8.
23. Siegel, J. Demographic aspects of aging and the older population in the United States, Series P-23, No. 59, 1982. In *America in Transition: An Aging Society,* Serial No. 99-B. Washington DC: U.S. Government Printing Office, 1985.
24. Irick C. Income of the new retired workers by social security benefit levels: Findings from the new beneficiary survey. *Soc. Secur. Bull.* 1985; 48(5): 7–15.
25. Ibid. pp. 12–13.
26. Schultz J H. *The Economics of Aging,* Third Edition. Belmont, CA: Wadsworth; 1985; 15–16.
27. Nursing Home Characteristics: Preliminary Data from the 1985 National Nursing Home Survey. Washington DC: National Center for Health Statistics Advanced Data, 131, March 27. 1987.
28. Stein, L I. The doctor–nurse game. *Archives of Gen. Psych.,* 1967; 16, 699–703.
29. Health Care Financing Administration, Division of National Cost Estimate. National health expenditure 1986–2000. *Health Care Financing Rev.,* Summer 1987; 8(4): 1–36.

3

Nursing Homes: Adding the Missing Ingredient

Joan E. Lynaugh and Mathy D. Mezey

Every patient in an acute care hospital can expect that his nurse cares for only three other patients. However, if he is transferred to a nursing home he may find that his nurse cares for as many as forty-eight other people, and that his nursing care may be less than fifteen minutes per day. This grim reality exists despite rising levels of acuity among nursing home admissions, increasing complexity of medical and nursing care requirements, and public apprehension about premature discharge of elderly persons from acute care hospitals.

Nurses and nursing care are essential to the nations' 19,000 nursing homes. Effective nursing and medical care for future nursing home residents depends on attracting skilled, qualified nurses to nursing home practice as well as sufficient funds to support more and better caretakers. But thoughtful health care planners recognize that more than money is needed. New approaches and new strategies with which to address the nursing home problem are necessary to assure that tomorrow's nursing homes will be safe and effective components of our health care system.

The Robert Wood Johnson Foundation Teaching Nursing Home Program experiment in long-term care nursing and medical practice offers one approach to the nursing home care dilemma. The project's premise is that nursing is the essential intervening variable.

Each experimental program was required to create a design that met the general objectives of the Teaching Nursing Home demonstration. These objectives were to: (1) find more effective ways to implement nurse and physician services for nursing home residents, (2) produce more nurses educated in gerontology, (3) improve the general standard of care in nursing homes, and (4) seek more effective ways to connect nursing home residents with other health care services in their communities. No specific model or strategy was required. Instead, the participants were encouraged to innovate approaches which they believed would yield measurably better care for residents and attract students. Each program was expected to develop a formal, legal affiliation between nursing school and nursing home that supported the overall objectives of the individual program and the national demonstration.

EXPERIMENT IN CARE

The five-year effort on the part of nursing school faculty and nursing home personnel is now yielding concrete data and useful insights on care problems in nursing homes. An overview of all the projects reveals two dominant strategies which address the patient care objectives of the experimental program. First, every project placed one or more clinical specialists or nurse practitioners in the nursing home to care for patients and work with staff. Second, every nursing home restructured its approach to delivering nursing care in some way. In retrospect, these two strategies proved vital and ultimately characterized the part of the project which focused on improving care. Because safe and effective care is at the heart of the teaching nursing home demonstration, each strategy warrants detailed explanation.

NEW NURSES

The new kinds of nurses introduced in these experiments are masters-prepared specialists, including geriatric nurse practitioners (GNPs), gerontological nurse specialists, and geropsychiatric nurse specialists. Their practice focuses on recognizing illness or dysfunction early; initiating diagnostic and therapeutic interventions promptly; providing accurate and comprehensive information on patient conditions to physicians; teaching other nurses and nurses aides strategies for preventing health care problems such as decubiti, dehydration, urinary track infections, or inappropriate medication use; and personally managing care for more complicated patients. Most of these new nurses work both as direct care providers and as consultants to other nursing personnel.

This strategy for improving patient care can best be explained through the words and experiences of the nurses themselves. First, they find their work captivating and challenging. "No day is ever the same here

. . . I almost never do the same things twice." Though nurses, physicians, health planners, and others have worried that bright young clinicians will be disenchanted by nursing home care, our observations have been just the opposite. The clinical problems posed by the elderly are complicated and highly varied. The expert nurse finds her knowledge, assumptions, and skills tested. Nursing home residents often develop problems of multifactorial etiology. As pioneer nurse gerontologist Doris Schwartz put it, elders' problems are, "due to multiple pathologies presented atypically, may be acute problems superimposed on chronic illness, may be inadequately reported by the patient, are partly iatrogenic, unpredictable in outcome, and complicated by defective mental status and difficult social circumstances."[1] A hallway conference in one of the teaching nursing homes echoed Schwartz's point: "We have to figure out if she is acting sick from the cancer or from her digitalis . . . or, from something else. Here is somebody whose potassium is low . . . and she is on digoxin. She can't tell us what she feels . . . so, let's get all our information together and see what else we need."[2]

Nurse specialists encounter many problems related to the mental status of the patients. In nursing homes, the incidence of cognitive impairment is estimated to be between 40% and 70%. Some estimates suggest that 80% of nursing home residents have a diagnosable psychiatric disorder. For instance, one often finds agitated, combative patients requiring restraint 24 hours a day. An expert psychiatric nurse clinician working in concert with family, staff, and physician, can sometimes free these patients from their restraints, reduce costs of care, and vastly improve the care environment by implementing planned interventions such as exercise, supervision, and documentation of behavior.

A significant task for each Teaching Nursing Home project was to clarify and, in some cases, reorganize clinical decision making in the nursing home. After five years of experimentation, most of the projects settled on a "shared decision making" strategy to manage stable and unstable chronic conditions, common acute conditions, complex acute conditions, and health promotion. Managing care includes selecting, ordering, and monitoring therapeutic modalities such as diet, ambulation, treatments, and medications. In some settings, the physician and the nurse shared in the decision making; in others, a multidisciplinary group was responsible. Other areas in which shared decisions were usually made include admission or readmission, assessment of the patient's status on admission, use of emergency rooms, hospitalization, referrals and discharge planning, although the nurse on the scene may be the primary decision maker.

Central to the process of change and clarification of clinical decision making, however, is the exchange of detailed and extensive information among the providers. As previously learned in ambulatory or critical care units, the nurse specialist enhances the specificity and the depth of clinical information passed from the nursing staff to the physician or other health providers.[3] Communications are more direct, with less deference and restraint. The confidence of the nurse practitioner or clinical specialist in her or his own clinical skills and knowledge supports expert recommendations and free exchange of ideas. All the masters-prepared nurses in the project report that encouraging staff nurses to collect data, organize information, and share research confidently with physicians and others is important. Experienced, talented nursing staffs had previously felt constrained or were bypassed and could not influence clinical decision making about their patients according to informal findings. Clarifying the clinical decision-making process, that is, making physicians, administrators, and nurses themselves aware of the crucial function of nursing information and judgment, enables staff nurses to share their knowledge in full where it counts.

NEW APPROACHES

Since no specific design or model was a prerequisite for any of the Teaching Nursing Home projects, each affiliated nursing home and school of nursing was free to focus on its own situation. Nevertheless, most of the projects elected to alter their care delivery in some way. Restructuring nursing service in the nursing home involved the most sweeping and difficult changes. Although designs varied, the two principles that guided change were commitment to continuity of nursing care and decentralization.

Essentially, the projects attempted to create a system in which a registered nurse has twenty-four hour, seven-day-a-week responsibility for a specific case load of patients. This system of patient care assignment currently is called the primary nursing model.[4] This model has obvious advantages over the functional system of assignment common in nursing homes. The functional system assigns a certain task, that is, medications, treatments, personal hygiene, to each nurse on duty, who then performs her or his assigned task for all the patients. The functional system of assignment is efficient and requires a small number of professional nurses: everyone is responsible for individual tasks, and no one is responsible for the individual patient except the nurse in charge. Such a system can work well in small facilities, but there are obvious drawbacks such as fragmentation, poor communication, and lack of accountability. These drawbacks are accentuated by rising levels of

acuity among patients, increased numbers of patients, larger proportions of patients with mental impairment, and high staff turnover.
The functional system of nursing assignment is also antithetical to nursing education which emphasizes the comprehension of all aspects of an
individual patient situation. It is not surprising that these experiments in
care involved changing the functional system. Given the limited number
of professional staff in the nursing homes, the challenge was to find
ways in which the system could be changed.

One intriguing example of the reorganization strategies tested by the
projects is the district nursing concept.[5] To assure the continuity of
nursing care needed for successful implementation of therapeutic regimens, one project reorganized residents and nursing personnel into
so-called "districts." A registered nurse was placed in charge of each
district. This district leader assessed, planned, implemented, and evaluated the care of the residents in conjunction with nursing assistants who
were directly accountable to the district leader. The district leader was
also responsible for continuity of care on evenings and nights even
though the leader practiced primarily during the day. The nursing
assistants sometimes rotated among the districts, but the district leader
retained a permanent district assignment. Thus, the registered nurse
had immediate responsibility for residents and for the work of nonprofessionals. Decentralization of authority allowed the registered
nurses to use their skills and knowledge to the best advantage for
individual residents and to assure continuity in nursing care for the
residents in her district.

In this district nursing project, the masters-prepared clinical specialist
served as clinical director. In this position, the clinical specialist established the standard of care, developed staff, guided complex patient
care management, and functioned as a primary caretaker. The masters-
prepared nurse used both line authority and professional influence to
achieve desired patient care outcomes. In this particular project, due to
improved continuity of care, clinical outcomes included a reduction in
dedubitus ulcers, reduced use of chemical/physical restraints, fewer
nosocomial infections, decreased use of enemas, fewer transfers to acute
care, and fewer residents who required total assistance with personal
hygiene.[6]

In addition to new approaches to organizing nursing care, some
Teaching Nursing Home projects focused on developing protocols or
standards of care. Several sites established interdisciplinary teams as a
means of implementing a comprehensive approach to care. These teams
made it possible to facilitate complex patient care plans and shared
decision making.

One Teaching Nursing Home site actually reorganized the entire administrative system for long-term care on its multilevel campus. The system brought together all components of long-term care—the nursing home, community health, acute rehabilitation, day care, and home care—under one nursing head so as to organize care around the patient.

WHAT THE EXPERIMENT IN CARE MEANS

Clearly the Teaching Nursing Home experiment relies on the assumption that introducing a clinical expert, in this case an expert nurse, is the most effective means of improving the quality of care for nursing home residents. The focus of nursing is to substitute for those things the person can no longer do for himself, to try to restore independence, to shore up personal resources, to alleviate suffering, and to help the dying. This professional focus ideally matches the care requirements of the institutionalized frail elderly.

Early measurements of the effectiveness of the clinical expert strategy, coupled with an emphasis on continuity and decentralization, suggest that clinical improvements do follow.[7] Studies of falls, incontinence, nutrition, and decubiti suggest that the clinical problems of patients in nursing homes are not necessarily inevitable.

Another aspect of the clinical expert strategy is the effect that the expert has on the behavior of others in the system. Early in the experiment, it became noticeable that students and staff imitated the actions and attitudes of the clinical specialist. Though not measured, this ripple effect of one nursing expert was demonstrated repeatedly, and it is difficult to estimate the real impact. Both staff and "new nurses" are aware of the reciprocal effect they have on one another. Staff appreciate the analytic, aggressive approach to clinical problems by the clinical specialist. In turn, the specialists appreciate the creative, sensitive care strategies of staff.

Less clear is the future of the relationship between the nurse practitioner or clinical specialist and the physician. Will the expert nurse substitute for the physician? Can these new nurses curtail unwarranted emergency room use or hospital admissions? The expert nurse represents a substantial added expense. Will the improvements in care and more effective use of resources offset these additional dollars? Though the answers are not yet certain, changing conditions in nursing homes will help forecast the outcome.

Higher acuity levels among admissions and complex patient case mix have become the norm in nursing homes. Traditional custodial care strategies are doomed to failure on these grounds alone. The institution-based expert is rapidly becoming essential. Teamwork between nurse and physician, analogous to that practiced in the intensive care units of hospitals, will be required. In the case of the nursing home patient, however, the nurse will be on-site and the physician will be primary based at a remote location. The chronicity of the nursing home population means that quality care must be maintained through mutually agreed upon plans, frequent communication, and shared decision making. Other necessary on-site disciplines include physical therapy and social work. In contrast, dentistry and podiatry are examples of disciplines that may operate from a remote base, involving episodic visits and consultations.

The Robert Wood Johnson Foundation Teaching Nursing Home Program has demonstrated that the expert nurse is the necessary ingredient in developing quality interdisciplinary services responsive to the complex problems of nursing home residents. The next step is to devise ways to make these expert nurses available to residents seeking quality care in nursing homes across the United States.

REFERENCES

1. Schwartz D. 1981; Personal communication.
2. Knaus W et al. An evaluation of outcome from intensive care in major medical centers. *Annals of Internal Medicine.* March, 1986 104 (3): 410–418. Prescott P, Driscoll, L. Nurse practitioner effectiveness, A review of physician–nurse comparison studies. *Evaluation and the Health Professions* (December, 1979) 2(4): 387–418. Feldman M. *Studies of nurse practitioner effectiveness. Nursing Research,* (September–October, 1987) 36 (5): 303–308.
3. Manthey M. Can primary nursing survive? *American Journal of Nursing* (May, 1988) 88 (5): 644–647. Joel L. The academic/nursing home duet: Care and teaching. Presented at The Robert Wood Johnson Teaching Nursing Home Northeast/Southeast Regional Consultative Conferences, Nov., 9, 1987, Danvers, MA and Jan. 28, 1988, Atlanta, GA.
4. Joel L, Johnson J. Increasing nurse authority shows results: Bergen Pines played role in curriculum changes. *AAHA Provider News,* April 15, 1988.
5. Ryan, S. See Chapter 6 of this volume for description of this project.
6. Henderson V. *The nature of nursing.* New York: The MacMillan Company, 1966: 15.
7. Bergstrom, N et al., "The Braden Scale for predicting pressure sore risk," *Nursing Research.* July–August, 1987; 36 (4); 205–210; Williams M. et al., Reducing acute confusional states in elderly patients with hip fractures *Research in Nursing and Health.* December, 1985; 8 (4): 329–346; Furstenberg A L & Mezey M, Differences in outcome between black and white hip fracture patients, *Journal of Chronic Diseases,* 1987; 40(10): 931–938.

4

Assessing the Effectiveness of Geriatric Nurse Practitioners

Robert L. Kane, Judith Garrard, Joan Buchanan, Sharon Arnold, Rosalie Kane, and Susan McDermott

Geriatric nurse practitioners (GNPs) have been shown to play an effective role in delivering primary care in nursing homes in at least two significant studies conducted over a decade ago.[1,2] More recently their role has been reaffirmed in a Veterans Administration study that focused on the training of housestaff but really relied on GNPs to deliver the nursing home care.[3] However, GNPs have not been widely introduced into active practice, at least in part because of restrictions in Medicare reimbursement policy under Supplemental Medical Insurance (Part B), which precludes direct payment for the services of a nurse practitioner not supervised on-site by a physician. Given this context, interest has shifted to exploring other ways in which the skills of geriatric nurse practitioners might be harnessed to improve nursing home care.

Beginning in 1975, with support from the W. K. Kellogg Foundation, the Mountain States Health Care Corporation in partnership with the schools of nursing at the University of Arizona, the University of California at San Francisco, the University of Colorado, and the University of Washington, developed a program of training for nurses to become nursing home-based geriatric nurse practitioners. The basic training

Acknowledgments: Funding for the evaluation of this project was provided by the Robert Wood Johnson Foundation and the Health Care Financing Administration, and by a grant to the Mountain States Health Corporation from the W. K. Kellogg Foundation.

model was adapted from earlier work in continuing education. Nurses with at least an R.N. but not necessarily a bachelor's degree, currently working in nursing homes were invited to apply for entrance into the program. Successful applicants had to have a sponsoring nursing home and a physician willing to serve as a preceptor.

Although there was some variation from school to school, the general training model featured four months of didactic instruction on the university campus and eight months of clinical work under the guidance of the physician preceptor at the sponsoring nursing home. Funds were available to defray the costs of the education and the preceptorship period, but the nursing home was expected to commit itself to hiring the graduate in a new role, that of a geriatric nurse practitioner.

The GNP was expected to serve as an interface with the physicians providing primary care to nursing home patients and a greater degree of clinical oversight to residents and inservice training to staff than was previously available in the nursing.home. In contrast to earlier mentioned studies, the GNP was an employee of the nursing home rather than an independent primary care provider. In this model, the nurse was not employed as a physician surrogate, but as a physician facilitator. Although the nurse related to one or more of the physicians serving the home's patients, the nurse did not supplant their activities. As a nursing home employee, the nurse was subject to the organization's administrative policies. The nurse was vulnerable, moreover, to frequent pressures to defray service costs by engaging in activities that would generate additional income or eliminate current expenditures (e.g., employee physicals, service to residents in related housing programs).

This program was implemented between 1975 and 1985 and was concentrated in eight western states. Because the program represented an important innovation in nursing care delivery, there was substantial interest in evaluating its effectiveness. The evaluation was begun in 1984 at the RAND Corporation and is still going on. It was partially transferred to the University of Minnesota where the principal investigator relocated. While RAND is performing the cost and use analyses, the University of Minnesota has responsibility for all other portions of the evaluation. Such an evaluation raises a number of important methodological and conceptual issues useful in understanding this project and others like it.

The research questions addressed in the evaluation thus far can be summarized as follows:

1. Do nursing homes with GNP's offer better quality of care as reflected in patient outcomes as well as measures of process?

Examples of improved outcomes include:
  better functional status
  greater satisfaction with care among patients and family
  more severe case mix on admission
  more discharges to the community
  less emergency room use
  lower incidence of decubitus ulcers
  lower incidence of urinary tract infections.
Examples of improved process measures include:
  closer medical attention
  less psychoactive drug use
  less restraints
  less urinary catheter use
  more appropriate care provided to patients with a series of tracer
  conditions.
2. Is the presence of a GNP associated with a cost saving to payors?
3. Is the presence of a GNP associated with a cost saving to the nursing home? What proportion of the GNP costs are recovered by the nursing home?
4. Do GNP effects differ by type of nursing home (i.e., size, ownership, patient mix, location)?
5. Do GNPs trained for nursing home work stay in that labor pool? Do they use their skills as GNPs? What factors currently impede the effective use of GNPs in nursing homes?
6. Do nursing homes with GNPs have a lower rate of citations from regulatory agencies?

The basic methodological design used in this evaluation to answer the research questions consisted of a comparison of data from matched pairs of homes. The experimental homes employed a GNP trained under the Mountain States program, the matched control homes did not employ a GNP.

Because this study relied on a quasi-experimental design that needed to separate the nursing home effect from that of the GNP, it was important to match nursing homes both with and without GNPs as closely as possible. This was done by identifying pairs of nursing homes. A target of 30 pairs was set as the minimum number required to provide an analysis of sufficient statistical power. Matching criteria included state (because of Medicaid regulations and issues of resource availability), bed size (including the proportion of skilled and intermediate beds), ownership (private, non-profit, public; chain or individual), hospital affiliation, occupancy rate, proportion of Medicare beds, and proportion of Medicaid beds. Given this stringent set of targeted conditions for matching, candidate nursing homes were sequentially contacted until the requisite number of matches could be obtained. As might be expected, the recruitment of control homes proved to be the rate limiting step. In several instances cooperation from one half of the pair could not be obtained, and in the absence of a suitable substitute the pair had to be abandoned. The 30 pairs of nursing homes were distributed, by state, as follows: Arizona (1 pair), California (10 pairs), Colorado (6 pairs), Idaho (2 pairs), Montana (1 pair), New Mexico (1 pair), Oregon (2 pairs), and Washington (7 pairs).

Because there are many characteristics of nursing homes that might affect the impact of a GNP on the nursing home and that we would not be able to select for, we also employed a pre/post design. In this way, we were able to control for differences between control and experimental homes that existed before the GNPs were employed when analyzing differences between the two types of nursing homes.

The research questions listed above required a wide range of data from a variety of sources. So that information from various sources could be combined to answer the research questions, time frames representing a preGNP period (before the GNP began work in the experimental nursing home), an interim period (while the GNP was undergoing her training), and a post-GNP period (after the GNP was in place and working in the experimental homes) were designated for each pair of facilities. Minor adjustments were made to accommodate each nursing home's fiscal year. Information on nursing home case mix, quality of care, resource use, cost, and role definition all required different data collection instruments. In addition to data obtained from written records such as nursing charts, financial statements, and state certificate and licensure records, data from three categories of subjects were gathered: (1) nursing home residents; (2) their families; and (3) professional staff, including GNPs, directors of nursing, and nursing home administrators.

The organization of the rest of this chapter follows the research questions described above. First, we describe the data collection methodologies used to collect information related to the quality of care questions: the retrospective chart review, the prospective patient interviews, and the family satisfaction questionnaire. Then, we describe the methodology relating to the cost component of the study. Various types of secondary data were collected for this section. Finally, we describe the data collection methodologies for the research questions relating to the larger organizational questions: how the GNPs fared in the nursing homes, whether they remain in that labor pool, and how the GNP affected the state regulatory agency perceptions of the nursing home in terms of the number of citations received.

RESIDENTS OF NURSING HOMES

Two approaches were used to assess case mix, quality of care, and patient resource use in the nursing home from the standpoint of the nursing home resident: (1) a retrospective record review, which examined separate samples of nursing home residents before and after the GNP, and (2) a prospective study, involving repeated interviews and observations of a sample of residents available only after the GNP was established.

The retrospective chart review allowed for the collection of a vast amount of information from experimental and control homes for both the pre- and post-GNP periods. However, we were cognizant that there might be systematic differences in the information available in the records kept. For example, the GNPs could result in better record keeping in the nursing home, without affecting the quality of care. If this were the case, differences in the chart reviews might not reflect real differences in patient status or quality of care. On the other hand, the GNP could have a significant impact on patients in areas that would not be reflected in the charts, e.g., on morale or satisfaction. For these reasons, it was decided that interviews with nursing home residents in a sample of homes participating in the study would provide valuable additional information. Since this evaluation was begun after the GNPs had been in place in the facilities, the interviews were conducted only after the GNPs were employed in the homes, but not necessarily coinciding with the post-GNP period used in the other data collection strategies.

Retrospective Record Reviews

In order to study changes in patient care characteristics and costs over time, repeated cross-sectional data were abstracted from the records of residents in 60 nursing homes, 30 with GNPs and 30 without.

A quasi-experimental design was used in this retrospective record review in which records were abstracted on a pre/post, experimental (GNP) comparison (non-GNP) group basis. Four separate samples of resident records were drawn randomly: pre-GNP, pre-non-GNP, post-GNP, and post-non-GNP. The study period for the pre-period component was one calendar year prior to the completion of training of the GNP in the nursing home and that of the post-period component consisted of the two years following completion of training of the GNP. Data for each pair of homes was taken from the same years. The years chosen for each pair of nursing homes was based on the completion of training of the GNP in the experimental home.

Resident records to be abstracted were randomly drawn from a list of all residents currently residing in the nursing home during the designated study periods. The pre-GNP study period was operationally defined as the year prior to the GNP's training (or arrival at the nursing home) and the post-GNP study period consisted of the two years immediately following the completion of training (including the preceptorship) or arrival at the nursing home. For each pair of matched homes, the times for the control home (the non-GNP home) were chosen to concur with those for the GNP home. In some cases minor adjustments were made to accommodate fiscal years to facilitate the cost component of the study. Residents were eligible for enrollment in the study only if they had been in the facility for at least six weeks during the study period and only if they were in skilled or intermediate beds, i.e., residents in residential apartments were not eligible. There were no other eligibility requirements, such as stratification by age, sex, race, etc.

Within each nursing home the design called for a total of 180 records to be randomly selected and abstracted: 60 records for the pre-GNP period and 120 for the post-GNP period. Within each of these two study periods, a greater proportion of residents who were admitted during the study period, compared with residents who had been in the nursing home prior to the beginning of the study period, were to be selected. Thus, in the pre-GNP study period, 40 of the 60 records to be reviewed in each nursing home were to be of admissions. In the post-GNP period, 96 of the 120 records reviewed in each nursing home were to be of admissions. Because the post-GNP period was two years long, the proportion of new admissions was higher to allow for the longer period of observation during which approximately half of these subjects would become second-year residents. The effective ratio of admissions to residents would thus be about 2:1 in both the pre-GNP and post-GNP periods.

We stratified sampling to differentiate between residents and admissions because it was hypothesized that the GNP would have a differential impact on the two types of patients. Improvements in the quality of care provided to patients as a result of the GNPs would most likely have a greater effect on the admissions, slowing their decline and possibly enabling them to be discharged back to the community.*

A retrospective record review instrument was specifically developed to abstract the residents' nursing home records for this study. Information collected from the charts included the functional status of the

---

*The admissions were not necessarily *new* admissions. We allowed patients to be sampled that had been in the facility before, had been discharged to the hospital, and were being admitted back into the nursing home.

patient at various times during the stay, use of select medications such as psychotropics and diuretics, use of resources such as physical therapy, occupational therapy, physician visits, nursing therapies provided, and assessment of the quality of care provided to patients with a series of tracer conditions such as diabetes, hypertension, and fever. It was designed to provide data to answer the research questions regarding process and outcome measures of quality of care and the cost of care to patients in the experimental and control facilities. All record abstractors were nurses ($N=38$) who had undergone a 5-day training program in the use of the instrument. The review form consisted of a 24-page, 67-item booklet for each record abstracted. The items were categorized as follows:

Demographic data about the resident.

Admission status—admission from, payor at time of admission, level of care, diagnoses upon admission

Discharge status—date of discharge if discharged before the end of the study period, status upon discharge, where discharged to, length of stay if discharged to a hospital, payor at time of discharge or end of study period, level of care at time of discharge, diagnoses at time of discharge.

Utilization of Health Care Services—number of physician visits, podiatry visits, dental visits; number of orders written by the physician for medication, laboratory/X-ray, special services, and nursing orders. Number of telephone orders for these services. Number of orders of these services written by the GNP. Number of physical therapy sessions, number of occupational therapy sessions, number of emergency room visits, with and those without tests, number of admissions to the hospital and length of stay for elective and emergency visits.

Tracer conditions for diabetes, congestive heart failure, hypertension, fever (up to three episodes), urinary incontinence, feeding behavior, and confusion.

Several items were measured at the time of admission (or the beginning of the study period) and upon discharge (or end of the study period): ambulation, transferring feeding, toileting, dressing, mental status, and behavior; visitors, visits by resident away from home.

The following variables were recorded for three two-week periods of time during the study period: immediately following admission to the nursing home, three months after admission, and prior to discharge or at the end of the study period:

Medication data—types of medication, dosage, total number of different drugs taken on a regular and a prn basis, and list of all drugs ordered on discharge from a hospital.

Nursing therapies for decubitus care, Foley catheter, bladder and bowel training, dressing changes, gait training, IV fluid, tube feeding ostomy care, restorative nursing, oral suction, fracture care, tracheostomy care, oxygen, prosthesis care, range of motion, pureed diets, and soft restraints.

Interviews of Nursing Home Residents

Information about the resident's perceptions of his or her care and an objective assessment of health and functional status by a health professional was gathered in a standardized, 1.5-hour interview. This interview was conducted in a subsample of 10 nursing homes, 5 GNP homes and 5 matched non-GNP homes. All interviewers were nurses who had undergone 10 days of training with the instrument, and all interviews were on a one-on-one basis with the resident. These interviews were done to supplement the information in the retrospective record reviews by providing a more comparable measure of patient status; however, because of the prospective nature of this instrument, the time frame of data collected with the two methods did not often coincide.

Each resident was interviewed up to 4 times during a 1-year period: the baseline interview, then 3-, 6-, and 12-months after this initial interview. With the exception of basic demographic data, the same interview protocol was used all 4 times. With few exceptions, the multiple interviews with each resident were conducted by the same nurse-interviewer. A total of 14 nurse-interviewers participated in this aspect of the study. All interviews were conducted on a posttest basis only, that is, after the GNP had become established in the nursing home.

The five pairs of nursing homes in the interview study were a subset of the 30 pairs of nursing homes which were the sites of the record review study. The five GNP nursing homes were chosen because they were deemed by the Mountain States Health Corporation to have the most stable GNP implementation. The non-GNP nursing homes were those originally matched to GNP homes in the overall study.

Within each of the 10 nursing homes, the sampling design called for a total of 100 residents to be randomly selected from a list of all residents currently residing in the home. Sixty percent of those interviewed were to be patients who were admitted to the nursing home after the beginning of the study and were interviewed initially within four weeks of their admission; 40% were residents at the beginning of the study. There was no stratification of subjects, e.g., on the basis of sex, race, age, payor, skilled nursing facility/intermediate care facility, etc. The actual number of interviews with a resident varied from one to four, depending on whether she or he was in residence at the nursing home when the next interview was scheduled, e.g., if a resident was discharged between the third and the sixth month, then two interviews were available: the baseline interview and the 3-month interview. If the resident was unavailable for an interview, then the resident was dropped from the study and no further interviews were conducted. Thus if a resident was temporarily discharged to the hospital at the time of the 6-month interview, but had returned to the nursing home by the 12-month interview, only two interviews were conducted, at baseline and 3-months. We expected the number of interviews to be reduced with each succeeding wave over the 1-year period due to discharge of residents from the nursing home, through death, discharge to community, hospital, transfer to another nursing home, etc. In the interest of protecting subject confidentiality, the residents randomly selected for this interview study were not the same individuals who were randomly selected in these ten nursing homes for inclusion in the retrospective record review study.

The interview protocol consisted of 149 items with 9 sections: (1) demographic data; (2) admission from/discharge to the nursing home, (3) cognitive domain; (4) satisfaction domain; (5) affective domain; (6) activities domain; (7) social interaction; (8) activities of daily living domain; and (9) pain and discomfort domain. Using factor analysis, factor scores were derived for the latter 7 domains in order to evaluate the resident's health status.

The interview protocol was developed and used initially in a previous study[4] of 212 residents in four nursing homes in the Los Angeles area in 1980–81.[5] The outcome measure derived from psychometric research of that study and factor analysis with the 212 residents can be summarized as follows:

Cognitive Domain. The cognitive domain consisted of a ten-item Mental Status Questionaire (MSQ)[6] and a comprehensive cognitive scale which consisted of a combination of the MSQ and scores from other cognitive items which included digit repetition, telling time, face-hand test, general orientation, and a coin recognition test. The comprehensive cognitive score was developed using factor analysis and helps to differentiate among residents, especially those at the lower end of the MSQ scale. The mean inter-interviewer reliability coefficients for the cognitive domain established in the previous study[5] were .89 for the MSQ and .84 for the comprehensive cognitive scale.

Satisfaction Domain. The satisfaction domain consisted of 14 items which measured the resident's satisfaction with various aspects of the care provided by the nursing home and with the nursing home environment. The mean inter-interviewer reliability coefficient was .88 for this domain.

Affective Domain. The affective domain contains 12 questions concerned with how often the resident felt a particular emotion during the past month. The factor analysis of this set of items clearly differentiated two groups of effect: those addressing positive emotions and those addressing negative ones. The positive effect scale had a mean reliability coefficient of .85, and the negative effect scale had a mean reliability coefficient of .62.

Social Domain. A social domain consisted of three scores: (1) an inside activities score based on the frequencies of participation during the past month in eight activities available at each nursing home, (2) an outside activities score based on two questions having to do with going outside the nursing home to people's homes, restaurants, entertainment, etc., and staying overnight at someone's home, and (3) a social contact score which focused on the frequency of contact with other residents, friends outside the nursing home, and family members outside the home, and the resident's assessment of the closeness of these interactions. Special attention was paid to whether the respondent had at least one person regarded as a confidant. The mean inter-interviewer reliability for the inside activities items was .70, and .59 for social interaction.

ADLs. Activities of daily living were evaluated on the basis of direct observations by the nurse interviewer and the resident's self-report of the ability to perform the following basic daily activities: bathing, toileting, transferring, dressing, feeding, remaining continent, and moving within bed. The first 6 items were developed by Katz and his colleagues[7]; the seventh item was added in the study of 4 Los Angeles nursing homes. These 7 items had a mean reliability coefficient of .80.

Pain and Discomfort Domain. A pain–discomfort scale was developed based on 6 items assessing frequency of pain and discomfort: aches, chest pain, shortness of breath, dizziness, itching, and headaches. The inter-interviewer reliability coefficient was .82 for this set of items.

Data from the Mountain States Project were factor analyzed, based on interviews with 712 residents for whom complete data were available. The factor analytic solutions showed no significant differences from the factor analytic solutions based on the 212 residents in the Los Angeles study. In fact, the factor scores were virtually the same for almost all variables.

NURSING HOME OBSERVATIONS

In order to observe the general conditions within each of the 60 nursing homes in the sample, four periodic inspections were completed in each home. The four observations were conducted at different points in time, two during the early phases of data collection and two during the later phases. Data collectors were instructed to observe the homes on four different days of the week and at different times of the day.

A posttest only, experimental comparison group design with repeated observations was used for this portion of the study. The data collectors were asked to report on the general status of patients within the home. The intent of this portion of the study was to note the overall living and care conditions of residents within the home. This was designed as an additional check on the quality of care provided in these homes which may not be reflected in the nursing home charts. The observation form recorded the proportion of the home's patients in each of the following categories; having indwelling catheters, being physically restrained, remaining in bed, not well groomed, not interacting with others, and requiring feeding.

FAMILIES OF NURSING HOME RESIDENTS

Telephone Interviews

In order to assess the satisfaction of family members (in the case of those residents who have family), each resident in the interview study (from five GNP nursing homes and five non-GNP homes) was asked to name the person he or she viewed as the key family member. The family member was interviewed on an individual basis by telephone up to three times during the one year, post-GNP study period: 3 months after the resident's enrollment in the study, 6 months, and 9 months.

A posttest only, experimental comparison group design was used with this prospective study of the opinions of family members. The time period was selected to represent duration long enough for an impression of care to have developed, yet not so long that a substantial number of residents would have been discharged. A brief telephone interview was used to assess the satisfaction of the relative with care the resident received while in the nursing home.

Sampling designs used in the resident interview study also were used in this interview study of family opinion. The subjects in this study were relatives of the residents in the five pairs of GNP and non-GNP nursing homes. If a nursing home resident was dropped from the study due to discharge from the nursing home, then the relative was also dropped as a subject for subsequent interviews in the family member satisfaction study.

The interview protocol consisted of a 12-item form in which the first 2 questions had to do with family member's relationship with the resident and whether or not he or she had visited the resident in the nursing home. If the resident had been visited, the interviewer asked the remaining 10 items which concentrated on the relative's assessment of quality of staff and care in the nursing home. A 5-point Likert scale was used which ranged from "Strongly Agree" to "Strongly Disagree."

COST ISSUES

Determining who benefits financially from the services of GNPs and the extent of the benefit is one of the major challenges facing this evaluation. Because nursing homes employ GNPs, the nursing home incurs the cost of employment. Even though the GNP role focuses on providing better patient care most nursing homes cannot bill directly for GNP patient care services or for any improvements in the quality of nursing care that result from GNP employment. Nursing homes may, however, benefit indirectly from the employment of GNPs, if by raising standards of care a nursing home attracts more patients or becomes more efficient. Unfortunately, these savings are much harder to measure.

By improving the quality of care that nursing home patients receive, GNPs may reduce the use of expensive medical care services outside the nursing home such as hospitalizations and emergency room visits. In this case, it is not the nursing home that receives the cost benefit but rather private and government payors. If government programs such as Medicare and Medicaid benefit from the employment of GNPs, then it would be advisable that these programs bear some of the costs incurred. Changes in the regulations regarding allowable reimbursable costs for these programs would then be warranted.

Medicare and Medicaid interact in complex ways to cover much of the costs of patient care for the populations being studied. Together government programs pay almost half of the costs of nursing home care. Medicare pays only a small portion of the costs of nursing home care, while Medicaid pays approximately 45% of these costs. Private payments, mostly from the patients and their families, pay for over half of nursing home costs. Most of the other medical care services used by the elderly and disabled, such as hospital care and physician services, are covered under Medicare. Medicaid frequently buys the supplemental medical insurance (Part B) services available under Medicare and is considered the second payor after Medicare for the poor.

If GNPs affect the progress of patients by increasing the proportion of patients who are discharged to the community, or by discharging patients sooner, Medicaid may benefit. The benefit is observable for patients who currently rely on Medicaid, but only potential for patients who would otherwise have exhausted their resources and become Medicaid eligible.

In the next section, we discuss methods for measuring the effect of GNPs on nursing home costs and revenues. The GNP's effects on the costs to the different payors follows. Realistically, we cannot hope to identify, quantify, and sort out all of these costs. We have attempted, at least, to describe the most important costs and to measure, where possible, the size of the effect resulting from the GNP influence.

NURSING HOME COSTS AND REVENUES

At the present time, a nursing home has relatively little ability to directly recover the added costs of employing a GNP, a more highly trained individual than the typical staff nurse employed in a nursing home. The presence of a GNP may, on the other hand, indirectly affect costs and revenues within the nursing home in a variety of ways: by attracting more patients, particularly more private patients, by reducing staff turnover, or possibly by increasing staff efficiency. As a consequence, it is important to measure the effect GNPs have on actual operating costs and revenues in the homes that employ them.

In order to determine the impact of GNPs on nursing home costs and revenues, data were abstracted from cost reports of the 60 participating nursing homes, 30 with GNPs and 30 without. Cost reports were requested for the fiscal years covering each nursing home's pre-GNP year, the 2 post-GNP years, and for the interim years, as well. The pre- and post-GNP years coincide with the fiscal year dates and were selected so that patient level data from the retrospective record review portion of the evaluation could be incorporated into the home level cost analysis.

Because the GNP training period (1 year) did not necessarily match the nursing home's fiscal year, the pre-period was selected as the first complete fiscal year preceding the training period and the post period began at the start of the first fiscal year following the training period. As a consequence, some nursing homes have 2 interim years while others have one.

The design is a cross-sectional, time series that spans the pre- and post-GNP time periods for both treatment (GNP) and control (non-GNP) homes. The unit of observation for these analyses is a nursing home fiscal year; data were collected on the interim years to complete the time series. There are 164 pre-GNP ($N=54$) and post-GNP ($N=110$) years and 88 interim years of data (3 pairs of nursing homes have no pre-GNP period and 5 pairs have only 1 post-GNP year). Most of the analysis will focus on the 164 pre- and post-GNP years of data.

Because the majority of the nursing homes in our sample participated in Medicaid, the Medicaid cost reports were selected as the primary source of cost data. These differ by state and change over time so data were aggregated to a consistent level and abstracted onto a common form. In some instances Medicaid cost reports were unavailable, either because the nursing home did not participate in Medicaid (2 Arizona homes and 2 state Veterans homes), or because copies of older reports could not be located and newer reports had not completed the various stages of processing. Where available, Medicare cost reports were substituted. Finally, a questionnaire designed to obtain parallel data was sent to nursing homes ($N=11$) where neither the Medicare nor the Medicaid cost reports were available. Every effort has been made to rely on a single source of data for each facility. Since the analyses will look at changes over time or will control for a facility specific component, a consistent reporting form within a facility was regarded as superior to the use of Medicaid cost reports for particular years and either Medicare cost reports or Parallel data questionnaire results for the remaining years.

The data collection time frame extends from 1977 through 1986, so careful consideration is given to adjusting properly all dollar figures to real dollar terms and to adjusting for regional price differences.

Validation of the data obtained from the various states' Medicaid cost reports will use Medicare cost reports. For fiscal years between 1977 and 1983, HCFA (Health Care Financing Administration) provided a full set of completed Medicare cost reports. Approximately half of the study's nursing homes participated in Medicare.

The analyses will include the following dependent variable: total *and* operating costs per patient day, patient care cost per patient day, revenue per patient day, and profits per patient day.

Independent variables obtained from the abstracted data include:

patient days by payor, occupancy rate, type of ownership, bedsize, number of admissions, state, urban/rural location, revenue sources, and types of ancillary services (laboratory, radiology, oxygen, physical, occupational, and speech therapies) offered. Year to year changes in these variables are also observed.

The home level analyses will incorporate patient casemix measures developed from the retrospective record review data. The incorporation of casemix data is important not only because casemix differences influence costs but also because GNPs are expected to affect the nursing home's casemix. In particular, it is hypothesized that homes with GNPs will accept and attract more severely ill patients. Information such as the distribution of patients by ADL scores; mental status; proportion of patients with behavioral problems, incontinence, or requiring special nursing therapies; average age of residents; percent requiring skilled care; and diagnostic mix will be important to the development of these measures. Careful attention will be paid to weighting the patient level data to create accurate casemix measures at the nursing home level. Since the sample size is limited, the final specification will be necessarily parsimonious.

A structured telephone survey of the 60 nursing home administrators provided additional information about the nursing home. This survey identified whether the home was part of a multilevel complex, if it had changed in size or ownership during the study, whether it was part of a chain, and the extent to which the home shared services with either other nursing homes or other patient care organizations under common ownership. These variables will also be included as explanatory variables in the home level analyses.

Summary nursing home classification measures developed in other segments of the evaluation will also be considered as explanatory variables in the cost function analyses. Particular candidates include categorizations based on (1) the extent to which the GNP role was fully implemented within the experimental homes, (2) citation frequency, and (3) attention to patient living conditions from the nursing home observation reports. Homes in which the GNP role was not fully implemented (for example, when the GNP assumed the responsibilities of the nursing home administrator or director of nursing as well as those of the GNP), may not achieve the same cost savings as homes with full-time fully operational GNPs. Homes with poor citation records or poor patient living conditions may have lower costs, but these lower costs may be the result of a failure to allocate sufficient resources in these areas.

Less structured telephone interviews were also conducted with the Medicaid agencies in seven states (except Arizona). These interviews provided information on the nursing home rate setting procedures in each state, any changes in the procedures during the study, allowable costs, staffing requirements, and the relative generosity of each program. Since the Medicaid program pays for around half of nursing home costs in most states, these interviews provide important background information on how states differ both initially, and in anticipated cost trends over time. This information allows us to anticipate, understand, and interpret differences across the states in this study.

Medicare Costs

While the Medicare program pays for only a very small portion of nursing home care, it pays for most physician and ancillary services delivered to nursing home patients as well as hospitalization costs for the elderly and the disabled, groups which comprise most of the nursing home population. GNPs may, in fact, alter the use of these other medical care services, particularly by reducing the need for hospitalization. Since the Medicare program currently does not reimburse GNPs directly for their patient care activities, it is important to identify cost savings that accrue to Medicare as a result of the GNP's activities.

Medicare Part A and Part B claims data are being obtained for Medicare patients from 12 nursing homes, 6 GNP homes, and 6 non-GNP homes. This claims data comes from HCFA's State and County Database and is available only for selected counties. As a result, 10 of the 12 homes are paired homes, 2 come from Oregon, 9 from California, and 1 from Washington. The sample includes approximately 1500 patients from the four sample groups pre-GNP, post-GNP, pre-non-GNP, and post-non-GNP. Data abstracted from medical records as part of the retrospective record review segment will be merged with claims data to provide comprehensive medical detail unavailable from analysis of claims data alone.

Short Medicare eligibility profiles are being extracted from Medicare's Health Insurance Master file through HCFA's HIPO (Health Insurance Print Out) system for these patients. The profiles specify Part A and Part B eligibility history, Medicare HMO enrollment data, cross-reference Medicare IDs, and dates of death.

Analysis of claims data allow us to look at whether GNPs have impacted on costs to Medicare. In addition to total expenditures, we plan to look at whether the costs of several components of care including hospital costs, nursing home based ancillary care, all outpatient ancillary care, and physician visit costs are affected. It is hypothesized that GNPs may actually increase the use of nursing home based ancillary care but will reduce costs overall.

Medicaid Costs

GNPs can affect Medicaid program costs in several ways: (1) through their impact on per diem nursing home costs, (2) by slowing the rate at which patients "spenddown" into Medicaid eligibility, that is, the Medicaid conversion rate, (3) by altering patient's expected length of stay, the rate of discharge to the community, and/or the mortality rate, and (4) by altering the use of other medical care services both for Medicaid patients and for patients who are both Medicaid and Medicare eligible. While we cannot measure the actual dollar impact on the Medicaid program in any of these areas, evaluation data will at least suggest the presence or absence of effects, the direction of the impact, and may provide insight into the magnitude of the effect as well.

Analysis of the effect of GNPs on per diem nursing home costs is discussed in the section on nursing home costs. Since the Medicaid program pays for much of the cost of nursing home care, and Medicaid reimbursement rates are based on per diem nursing home costs, the effect of any significant savings in per diem costs would eventually accrue, at least in part, to the Medicaid program. (Through restrictions on allowable costs, Medicaid programs have methods to protect against cost increases in GNP homes.)

If GNPs effectively reduce hospital and/or other medical care use, private patients conserve their resources and will not "spenddown" into Medicaid eligibility as rapidly as would otherwise have occurred. Detecting true differences in the spenddown rates is not possible with available evaluation data. This would require information on patients' financial assets and income. We can, however, test whether the spenddown rates in the post-GNP years in GNP homes have been reduced from pre-GNP year levels when compared to non-GNP homes. Such findings, while not conclusive, would clearly suggest that GNPs affected spenddown rates. The key assumption, although untestable, which underlies this analysis is that the *real* financial position of the average patient admitted to each nursing home did not change between the two periods.

GNPs can potentially affect the probability of discharge to the community, the mortality rate, and the expected lengths of stay for patients in each category. To the extent that GNPs significantly alter traditional patterns of nursing home use, we can estimate the nursing home per diem costs associated with GNP and non-GNP patient patterns. This information when combined with data on spenddown rates would allow us to infer potential additional savings to Medicaid.

Finally, if the analysis of Medicare claims data indicate that GNPs impact on Medicare costs for patients who are both Medicare and Medicaid eligible, it is expected that Medicaid costs will be affected as well.

The impact on Medicaid costs would be much smaller since Medicaid pays only admissible costs left unpaid by Medicare. For patients with only Medicaid eligibility, the full effect of altered patterns of medical care use would accrue to the Medicaid program. While we will not be able to determine the precise dollar impact, again the evaluation data allow us to determine the direction of the effect and may provide boundaries on the magnitude.

Patient Level Medical Care Use and Imputed Expenditures

In order to determine the impact of the full complement of GNPs on the costs and use of medical care for all patients, we analyzed use data obtained from the retrospective record review portion of the evaluation. Since the dollar is a convenient metric for equivalencing the use of different services, data on the use of medical services from the retrospective record reviews will be assigned prices and aggregated to determine how GNPs impact on total expenditures. The use of imputed prices avoids problems of converting to constant dollar terms and factoring out regional price differences inherent in analyses of actual cost and claims data.

Since these data are derived from the retrospective record review component of the evaluation, the quasi-experimental design with pre-post-treatment and control groups is replicated in this section as well. The sample includes approximately 9200 patients randomly drawn from the four groups: pre-GNP, pre-non-GNP, post-GNP, and post-non-GNP.

In addition to the measure of imputed expenditures, we will look at the use of different medical care services including hospitalizations, emergency room visits, physical and occupational therapy, and physician and podiatry visits. We will look both at counts of the use of these services and at the probability of use.

PROFESSIONAL STAFF PERSPECTIVES: GERIATRIC NURSE PRACTITIONERS (GNP), DIRECTORS OF NURSING (DON), NURSING HOME ADMINISTRATORS (NHA)

Telephone Interviews: GNP, DON, NHA

The nurse practitioner's role as a staff member of a nursing home is relatively new. In fact, our sample of 30 homes constitutes a large proportion of the nursing homes in the United States known to employ GNPs directly. The experiences of GNPs and of key persons in their work environment is important to capture because such data helps to pinpoint specific ways that the GNP role has been formulated and the factors that influenced those formulations. A case study methodology that incorporated a series of interlocking telephone surveys was used to examine the GNP's role and its implementation. Specifically, individual telephone interviews were conducted with the GNPs (N=30), the direct-ors of nursing (*N*=27), and the nursing home administrators (*N*=29) in the GNP nursing homes. The purpose of these interviews was fourfold: to find out the extent to which the GNP role had been implemented, to learn what might facilitate or impede the development of the GNP role, to understand what the GNP perceived to be the resident outcomes of GNP care, (and to examine the extent of congruence among these three distinct professional roles in each facility regarding the GNP role and effectiveness. Since one of the GNPs served in the dual role of GNP and nursing home administrator, only 29 administrators were interviewed; likewise, 3 of the GNPs also served as directors of nursing (DON), hence, 27 DONs were interviewed.

The design used with these three groups of professional staff was the three-group, posttest, single interview. Each subject was interviewed once by telepgone on an individual basis. All GNPs, DONs, and nursing home administrators (NHA) in the sample of 30 nursing homes with GNP staff were included in this part of the study.

The interview required approximately one hour and was based on a semistructured protocol. The GNP protocol consisted of a 19-item form organized around four major categories: (1) background information about the GNP, (2) the extent of GNP role implementation in direct patient care for residents and direct nonresident care such as staff physicals, administrative tasks, quality assurance, and research, (3) GNP perception of effectiveness and potential impact of GNP role on resident outcomes, and (4) GNP relative satisfaction and factors that may have facilitated or impeded implementation of the GNP role in the nursing home. The DON and NHA protocols each consisted of 9 items which covered the same broad topics as the GNP form. In addition, the DON protocol specifically asked about the relationship between the GNP and the DON—a description that was elicited by the question posed to the GNP regarding factors that facilitated and impeded im-plementation of the GNP role. The DONs also were asked how they would design the GNP role now, based on their experience over the past several years.

Work Histories of GNPs

In order to more fully examine the GNP in the role of nursing home staff, a study was conducted toward the end of the post-GNP data collection period of the work histories of control GNPs in this study compared to GNPs who graduated from the same educational programs during the same time period. We were particularly interested in studying the extent to which the experimental GNPs remained in the GNP role. To broaden the base of work histories and to provide a point of comparison, we also followed the classmates of the GNPs in our sample.

The methodological design was a two-group, pre-post-GNP training period based on subject's recall. All experimental GNPs ($N=30$) in this study were compared with all other graduating GNPs ($N=72$) from the same university-based GNP programs during the same period of time. The list of all graduates from 1977–86 of the GNP university-based programs in Arizona, California, Colorado, and Washington was obtained. Each of these graduates was mailed a 5-page questionnaire, with two mailed follow-up letters and a telephone follow-up for nonrespondents.

The work history questionnaire focused on demographic characteristics, educational preparation and professional experience prior to the GNP program, institutional sponsorship, and title and duties of professional positions before and after the GNP training.

CITATIONS OF NURSING HOMES

One of the areas in which the presence of a GNP might have a positive impact is review by regulatory agencies. The annual certification inspections can result in citations of various degrees of stringency for items not found to be in compliance with regulations. Although a facility's record of citations may not accurately reflect the quality of its care, attention to this index is important because: (1) these citations represent the official status of a home, (2) they are available to the public as a measure of the home's quality, and (3) they are also of great concern to the nursing home operators. If the presence of a GNP can improve the home's performance in the eyes of the regulators, the home may be motivated to employ such an individual. This study consisted of a comparison of citation history in regulatory review records for the GNP nursing homes and the non-GNP homes in order to examine changes in the frequency and nature of citations associated with the presence of GNPs in a home.

The unit of analysis in this study was the nursing home. A quasi-experimental design based on retrospective record review of pre-post-GNP study periods for the experimental (GNP homes) and comparison (non-GNP homes) groups was employed. All GNP ($N=29$) and non-

GNP (*N*=29) homes were included in this study. Under the aegis of the Mountain States Health Cooperative, citation records for nursing homes with SNF beds were requested from the state regulatory agencies in the eight states. (One pair of nursing homes in New Mexico did not have skilled nursing facilities.)

A copy of the pre-1986 HCFA form for each of the SNF facilities was requested. This form includes SNF criteria (designated by HCFA as F codes) which consist of 18 conditions of participation, one of which is nursing services. The analysis of these data from this aspect of the regulatory system focused on types of citations across the 18 conditions and a more in-depth look at the severity of patient-related citations of standards within the Nursing Services condition.

GNPs' PERCEPTIONS OF IMPACT, EFFECTIVENESS, AND BARRIERS

Although the results of the evaluation are not yet available, some sense of the extent of outcome can be derived from responses of the GNPs to interview questions regarding perceptions of their role and its impact. Table 4.1 shows the relative emphasis the GNPs ascribed to different aspects of their work. The areas most often cited were those that facilitated and complemented the work of the physicians such as performing physical examinations on patients or giving acute care, assisting with physician visits, performing patient assessments, monitoring or ordering drugs and laboratory tests (with countersignatures), and making rounds on patients. However, the GNPs also did a number of other tasks as well. Some of these activities, listed in Table 4.2, may be viewed as appropriate extensions of the GNP role, while others threaten to detract from the primary focus of that activity, perhaps motivated by a pressure to generate additional revenue for the nursing home in order to defray the costs of the GNP's salary.

When GNPs were asked about the effects they thought they had achieved, the predominant pattern of responses again pointed to close links with the physicians. As shown in Table 4.3, they cited reduced hospital use, better working relationships with physicians, reduced pain and discomfort and improved function among patients, and an ability to admit sicker patients to the nursing homes.

The GNPs also noted some barriers to their ability to use the skills they had acquired. When they were asked to name these without any prompting, the list shown in Table 4.4 emerged, headed by physicians and nurses. However, in response to a standardized list of potential problems, they cited more often limitations imposed by regulations and

TABLE 4.1   Areas Where GNPs Perceived They Had Substantial Emphasis

Activity	Percent of GNPs believing it got substantial emphasis
Episodic physicals/acute care	90
Assist physician visits	80
Routine physical assessment	77
Monitor/order drugs	73
Order lab tests	70
Make rounds	67
Critical care	60
Rehabilitation	43
Counseling	40
Serve on call	17

TABLE 4.2   GNP Activities Other than Service to Nursing Home Patients

Activity	Percent of GNPs performing it
Inservice education	80
Quality assurance	77
Administration/supervision	63
Minor health care to staff	47
Care to independent living residents	43
Pre-employment/annual staff physical	37
Counseling staff	27
Research	23
Home evaluations/discharge planning	13

TABLE 4.3   Areas Where GNPs Perceived They Had a Substantial Effect

Area	Percent of GNPs perceiving substantial effect
Reduced acute hospitalizations	63
Better physician relationships	60
Reduced pain/increased comfort	57
Improved physical functioning	53
Sicker case mix	50
Improved cognitive functioning	30
Improved social functioning	27
More discharges to comunity	20

**TABLE 4.4 GNPs' Unprompted Perceptions of Obstacles
to their Effective Performance**

Perceived barrier	Percent of GNPs perceiving it
Physicians	33
Nurses	30
Working only part-time as a GNP	23
Not enough time/too much work	23
Role confusion	20
Administrators	10
Budget pressures	7
Reimbursement	7
Regulations	7
Insufficient pay	3
Poor equipment	3

pressures created by the system of reimbursement (or more accurately the lack of direct reimbursement for their services).

IMPLICATIONS

The problem of improving the quality of care in nursing homes is a national one. Within the health care field, improvement in the quality of health care and the provision of cost-effective care constitute a major, ever-growing concern, especially as the proportion of older Americans in our population increases. National and state legislatures, county commissions, and city councils are continually faced with issues of nursing home care. While their concerns may lie equally with escalating costs and the quality of care, there is a growing consensus that "something must be done." Within the nursing home industry, there are abundant problems that relate to quality improvement. The industry is heavily regulated by national and state agencies. While regulations have been necessary, their sometimes arbitrary implementation has fostered antagonistic, adversarial roles based primarily on money—what services will be payable, for how long, for whom, and under what conditions. Ostensibly, regulations are related to quality and accountability, but the tenor of the conversations is one of suspicion. It is this distrust that too frequently dominates the thinking of owners, administrators and public agency heads, not a concern for quality improvement. Long-term care administrators are genuinely and properly concerned with inflationary costs. When legitimate business interests are confronted by restricted reimbursement, economy of effort becomes essential. While no one would challenge the need for efficiency and economy, there have been real and adverse effects. In general, the skill level of nursing home employees is not high. Staff turnover is very high, sometimes in excess of 100% per year. Both of these problems are thought to be due to the low salaries of nursing home employees, most probably a direct result of cost control measures.

Proposals to change the current nursing home situation must recognize present problems. The nursing home does not enjoy high status either among the general public or among the professions. It is difficult to get physicians to attend their patients there; it is hard to recruit good nurses to work there. The GNP represents one attractive means to improve the provision of primary care to nursing home patients. Recent legislation has extended Part B reimbursement under Medicare to physician assistants. GNPs similarly should be covered.

Within the field of nursing there are continuing debates about the appropriate preparation of GNPs. The model tested here was derived from the period when continuing education was the mainstay of GNP training. As with nurse practitioners in general, the continuing education model has given way to a master's level preparation, which should produce an even more able graduate. However, as with any professional training, close attention must be directed to the importance of environment. There is good reason to believe that the situation in which a professional practices may have more to do with determining performance than formal preparation.[8] Our preliminary results indicate the possibility that GNPs employed by nursing homes may not be in a strong enough position to make the requisite changes in the practice environment. Pressures from administration to produce revenue may take priority over quality improvement goals. The GNP may be in a stronger position to influence care as an outside provider, working in concert with physicians, but maintaining a status independent of the nursing home.

Another force that can inadvertently thwart potential contributions of the GNP is the regulatory system. Designed to respond to the low level of care extant at the implementation of Medicaid, regulations can become serious impediments to innovation. To the extent that they emphasize process measures, regulations tend to rely on professional orthodoxies that have no empirical basis. As a new concept, the GNP represents a potential form of heresy, at a time when reformation is sorely needed. The GNPs' observations that regulators often restricted their activities directly or indirectly and the insensitivity of the citation system to real changes in quality of care point to a need to modify the regulatory process to assure that it will not hinder the evolution of creative change.

In this, and previous quality improvement projects, it has been clearly demonstrated that nursing homes want to be involved; committed nurses want an opportunity to secure advanced knowledge and skill development; and nursing home residents can tell the difference when a GNP is on staff. The focus of this evaluation has been to document and study the specific impact of the GNP as a nursing home staff person on the quality of care of residents and the cost effectiveness of this care. As described above, the subject, and therefore the study, are complex, using multiple outcome measures under different methodological conditions which focus on a variety of people affected by and effecting the quality of nursing home care and costs.

REFERENCES

1. Kane RL, Jorgensen LA, Teteberg B, Kuwahara J. Is good nursing home care feasible? *J Amer Med Assoc* 1976; 235: 516–519.
2. Master RJ, Feltin M, Jainchill J, Mark R, Kavesh WN, Rabkin MT, Turner B, Bachrach S, Lennox S. A continuum of care for the inner city: Assessment of its benefits for boston's elderly and high-risk populations. *N Eng J Med* 1980; 302: 1434–1440.
3. Wieland D, Rubenstein LZ, Ouslander JG, Martin SE. Organizing an academic nursing home. *J Amer Med Assoc* 1986; 255: 2622–2627.
4. Kane RL, Bell R, Riegler S, Wilson A, Kane RA. Assessing the outcomes of nursing-home patients. *J Geront* 1983; 38: 385–393.
5. Kane RL, Riegler S, Bell R, Potter R, Koshland G. *Predicting the Course of Nursing Home Patients* (Report N-1786-NCHSR). Santa Monica, CA: Rand Corporation; 1982.
6. Pfeiffer E. A short portable mental status questionnaire for the assessment of organic brain deficit in elderly patients. *J Amer Geriatr Soc* 1975; 23: 433–441.
7. Katz S, Ford A, Moskowitz R, Jackson B, Jaffee M, Cleveland M. The index of ADL: A standardized measure of biological and psychosocial function. *J A Med Assoc* 1963; 195: 914–919.
8. Moscovice IS. The influence of training level and practice setting on primary care provided by nursing personnel. *J Community Health* 1978; 4: 4–14

5

Reimbursement Options for Encouraging Geriatric Nurse Practitioner Services

Mathy D. Mezey and William Scanlon

Expenditures for nursing homes are of significant concern to both consumers and government agencies. In the past 20 years, they have come to represent 8.5% of the total bill for national health care, or $32 billion for 1986. By the year 2000, nursing home expenditures could double their 1982 level, making spending for nursing homes the fastest growing cost in health care.[1,2]

Discussions of policy regarding payment for care in nursing homes focus on direct cost to patients and the drain on public dollars, specifically state Medicaid budgets. Approximately 48% of the cost for nursing home care comes from out-of-pocket expenditures by patients which either cover the cost of care for the entire nursing home stay or, more commonly, cover costs until resources are exhausted, i.e., patients "spend down" private resources and thus become Medicaid eligible. Medicaid, the major federal/state program identified with nursing home care is responsible for 49% of all nursing home payments.[3] In many states, over 50% of the total Medicaid budget is spent on the less than 5% of elderly who are nursing home patients.[4]

In contrast to Medicaid, the impact of severe limitations on reimbursement by Medicare to nursing homes and its effect on costs and quality of care is rarely discussed. The Medicare program has been so successful in avoiding payment for stays in nursing homes that it is almost a footnote in the health policy debate regarding nursing home spending. It can be argued, however, that the Medicare costs associated with nursing home care have been seriously underestimated and that Medicare, therefore, should focus more attention on the appropriate role of nursing home care in an efficient health care system.

A potential way to reduce Medicare costs without threatening quality is to discourage use of expensive hospital and out-patient services when equivalent care can be safely provided within the nursing home. Until recently, the lack of nursing home personnel capable of providing such care precluded making such a recommendation. Recent findings from the Robert Wood Johnson Foundation (RWJF) Teaching Nursing Home Program (TNHP), along with data from other demonstration projects and practice arrangements, have shown that geriatric nurse practitioners (GNPs) markedly increase the capability of nursing homes to care for sicker patients. Establishing ways to fund employment of GNPs has the potential to both improve care and decrease overall Medicare Part A and Part B costs for nursing home patients.

MEDICARE EXPENDITURES FOR NURSING HOME CARE

Given the magnitude and growth of expenditures, it comes as no surprise that public programs have made serious efforts to control spending in nursing homes. Long before the popularity of cost containment with respect to hospitals, Medicare and Medicaid instituted payment and coverage rules to limit the expenditures in nursing homes. Medicaid's efforts have undoubtedly reduced spending from that it would have been. However, because of Medicaid's role as the "funder of last resort" and the genuine need for nursing home care by significant numbers of elderly, Medicaid nursing home expenditures remain sizeable.

In the first years of the Medicare program, both utilization and expenditures in nursing homes far exceed anticipated levels. The program responded by restricting coverage to posthospital, skilled nursing or rehabilitative care only, and nothing for custodial care.[5] The vigor with which these impositions were employed and the animosity produced in nursing home operators who would rather not deal with the program has significantly limited direct payment to nursing homes through Medicare. In 1986, Medicare spent about $600 million for nursing home stays, accounting for only 1.6% of the revenue in nursing homes.[6] Medicare restrictions extend beyond the cost of nursing home care itself to the costs of physician visits to nursing home patients. To limit potential abuses—for example, making perfunctory visits to multiple patients on a single trip or seeing individual patients more frequently than needed—physician reimbursement is restricted to visits at specified intervals for routine medical care, to recertify the patient's need for nursing home care, and to medical emergencies.

The potential ineffectiveness of these strategies in containing Medicare costs for nursing home patients is obvious. Medicare loses when nursing home patients are hospitalized for treatment that might be provided in the nursing home. The most discussed aspect has been the additional hospital expenditures that result when Medicare patients are forced to remain hospitalized because no nursing home is willing to admit them.[7] Moreover, Medicare pays virtually all of the bill for the roughly 25% of nursing home patients hospitalized each year.[8] Even modest reductions in hospitalization could yield considerable savings to Medicare and, simultaneously, fund improved care in nursing homes. While hospital stays have always been expensive, under the new Prospective Payment System (PPS) Medicare is obligated to pay a fixed hospital rate irrespective of length of stay. A preventable admission from a nursing home invariably involves a shorter stay and less resource use than average, but now Medicare pays the full Part A hospital costs of an average admission in addition to the Part B physician costs, which can be significant.[9]

Medicare Part B costs are rarely included when calculating Medicare expenditures for nursing home patients. Medicare pays for physician visits to nursing home patients irrespective of whether the nursing home stay is paid for by Medicare, Medicaid, or privately. Federal regulations mandate that physicians visit (i.e., recertify) intermediate care (ICF) patients every 60 days and skilled (SNF) patients every 30 days.[10] Medicare Part B costs accrue from visits to recertify patients for continued nursing home placement, from episodic physician visits to nursing homes for routine medical care, or when patients experience acute but nonspecific health status changes. In addition, many nursing homes patients receive physician care in physician's offices or emergency rooms. Estimates indicate one-third of all nursing home patients are seen annually in an emergency room.[11] An unknown fraction of this physician care could readily be provided within the nursing home. In 1980, the cost to Medicare of physician visits in Michigan nursing homes was estimated at $2.4 million. Using this figure as a guide, a conservative estimate of costs to Medicare Part B for physician care in nursing homes in 1986 would be $122.3 million.[12]

Rising acuity among nursing home patients will surely further increase overall Medicare Part B expenditures, especially since those using nursing homes are older and sicker than the general population over 65. Characteristics of nursing home patients include an average of 12.8 diagnoses,[13] frequent use of medications (often more than 5),[14] and serious mental impairment in at least half the population.[15] With a more complex case mix, nursing homes increasingly will provide technologically intensive "sub-acute" care, terminal care, and long-term care for patients with multiple physical and mental health problems.

In light of these projections, strategies to reduce Medicare's per unit cost of medical care for nursing home patients while at the same time providing care within nursing homes substituting for more expensive outside services, should be welcome.

GNPs IN NURSING HOMES

It is well recognized that adult nurse practitioners provide primary care safely, effectively, and at reasonable cost.[16,17]

Performance quality: Studies show that nurse practitioners can provide primary care safely and as effectively as physicians. The quality of medical services provided by nurse practitioners is at least comparable to the quality of services provided by physicians. In some instances, nurse practitoners show superior quality in areas of symptom relief, diagnostic accuracy, and patient satisfaction. It has also been shown that the time spent by a nurse practitioner is greater (up to 65% more) than the time spent by a physician per visit. Nurse practitioners see 60% as many patients per hour as do doctors. The rationale for the additional time is the area of patient education and counseling, however, this area has not been recognized as reimbursable.

Productivity: The OTA review centers around the difficulties in measuring productivity in economic terms when applied to nurse practitioners. Structural constraints such as what nurse practitioners do as opposed to what they can do come into play. However, in a review of 15 studies concerning delegation of tasks, it was determined that 75 to 85% of adult care could be delegated to a nurse practitioner. Accounted for in this calculation are the extent to which tasks are delegated from a physician to a nurse practitioner, the amount of time it takes a physician or nurse practitioner to perform this same task, and the impact of the introduction of nurse practitioners on physician behavior.[18]

In looking at the impact of physician extenders working in consort with physicians in practice settings, Greenfield found that physician time required for consultation was 92% less than the time the physi-cian would spend treating the same clinical problem. Productivity levels comparing an M.D./nurse to an M.D. nurse/practitioner found a 25.8% increase. Estimates of increases in productivity in physician practices after the introduction of a nurse practitioner range from 20% to 90%. To quote the OTA review "The greatest productivity increases come when the nurse practitioner has primary responsibility for a subset of patients and when triage is performed by the nurse practitioner's referring "up" to the physician rather than the physician delegating routine medical problems "down" to the NP."[19] This is the most prevalent mode of NP/MD consultation in nursing homes.

Cost estimates: Increased physician extender participation can result in cost savings between 19 to 49% of total primary care provider costs. In the OTA review of employment costs of doctors or nurse practitoners, it was determined that the (1975) median hourly wage for a physician extender was about $6 compared to $24 for a physician. A CBO study comparing the cost of a physician extender with a physician found that if salary and the supervisory time of the doctor are included in the estimate, the hourly cost of a nurse practitioner is between one third and one half of physician costs ($12/hour compared to $24/hour).

Findings from recent studies show that GNP care to nursing home patients is similarly effective.[20,21,22,23] In over two-thirds of the eleven TNHP sites GNPs play a pivotal role in implementing project objectives. Specificially, GNPs provide: comprehensive admission and ongoing assessment; early recognition, diagnosis, and treatment of illness through routine surveillance; instructing licensed nursing staffs and nurses' aides on strategies to prevent decubiti, dehydration, urinary tract infections, and inappropriate use of medications, all of which are major sources of nursing home morbidity and hospital transfer. Moreover, GNPs enhance the facility's capability of managing patients with increased levels of complexity.

Rather than decreasing physician involvement in the care of nursing home patients, GNPs complement the physician role and increase physician efficiency. GNPs facilitate physician access to timely and accurate information, thus, decreasing overall time spent on unnecessary activities. By indicating when telephone consultation is sufficient, GNPs decrease unnecesary visits by physicians, emergency room transfers, and hospitalizations.

Findings from the "Nursing Home Connection," (Massachusetts 1115: Case Managed Medical care for Nursing Home Patients), a HCFA waiver program,[24] illustrate the cost effectiveness of case managed care for individual and groups of nursing home patients. In 1986, 2,000 patients in 100 nursing homes were served by 16 participating provider teams consisting of physicians, NPs, and physician assistants. Seventy-five percent of nonphysician participants were nurse practitioners. Under the program's waiver provisions, restrictions are lifted on the number of allowable monthly visits. Billable visits include mandatory 30- and 60-day recertifications, and visits to evaluate and manage acute and chronic illness. In the four years of the program, Federal savings were projected at more than $2,600,000, with state savings projected above $314,000, for a total program savings of $2,286,000. Number of visits to the nursing home totaled approximately 1.5 visits per month. The cost of increased visits was offset by reductions in emergency room use and hospitalizations, which declined by approximately 25% for an estimated savings of over $2,000,000 per year.

Further recognition of the potential of GNPs to improve quality of care and reduce costs is reflected in the increased employment of GNPs in HMOs and life care communities. HMOs are at financial risk for avoidable hospitalizations. Group Health of Puget Sound, which uses GNPs to make independent nursing home visits for problems that arise between physician visits, has applied for a Medicare waiver to permit GNPs to perform recertification as well.[25] GNPs employed by Kaiser Permanente of Oregon visit nursing home patients between physician visits to provide acute, chronic, and podiatry case; data are being accumulated regarding the number of hospitalizations prevented as a result of this intervention.[26]

Based on the financial structure of life-care communities it is advantageous to limit nursing home utilization by maintaining independence of residents. GNPs employed in life-care communities see residents for yearly physicals and for acute and chronic illness management. They treat residents in their residential quarters to avoid unnecessary transfers to the more expensive nursing home facility, and they see patients in the nursing home to facilitate early transfer back to independent living.[27,28]

Despite these demonstrated clinical benefits and cost savings, the current structure of the nursing home market discourages nursing homes from employing GNPs. Funded projects such as the TNHP underwrite GNP employment. To maintain the GNP role beyond the project period requires that nursing homes find revenues to cover GNP costs. Because many homes face restrictions on Medicare or Medicaid reimbursements, sustained GNP employment could be accomplished only by foregoing some other expense or by using revenues from private patients. Incentives are not strong and may not exist at all for nursing homes to find these revenues. Moreover, while GNPs enable a nursing home to handle acute problems and to deal with a more complex casemix, such a caseload can increase other nursing home costs. Neither Medicare nor Medicaid reimbursement may increase in response, so that profits will be squeezed rather than enhanced. If the potential for GNPs to improve care and decrease costs is to be fully realized, it is critical to develop funding options to expand their participation in nursing homes.

The OTA report concludes:

> Innovative approaches to improving the care and reducing the cost associated with nursing homes need to include modifications of regulations concerning visit limitations and changes in other Medicare and Medicaid regulations that limit the role of nurse practitioners in nursing homes.[29]

REIMBURSEMENT OPTIONS

Reimbursement of the GNP under Medicare Part B for services currently reimbursed physicians could significantly improve quality and access to care while potentially being cost saving.

According to the OTA report:

> Except when more intensive care can be substantiated, the number of physician visits to nursing homes is limited under the Medicare program. Extending coverage to GNPs, therefore, might not increase the cost attributable to nursing home visits for third parties payors, assuming payment levels are the same or lower for nurse practitioners as for physicians.[30]

Amendment of Medicare law (Public Law 99–509) in 1986 to authorize physician assistants, under the supervision of a physician, to recertify patients in skilled and intermediate nursing facilities provides precedence for such reimbursement. A bill to reimburse GNPs in a similar fashion for comparable services has been introduced in the current Congress.[31] Medicare Part B reimbursement would encourage GNP employment by physicians and HMOs, and would allow GNPs to contract directly with physicians and homes to provide care to nursing home patients. Alternatively, GNPs could supply physician substitute services to nursing home patients as independent practitioners similar to physical therapists, or contract with physicians to see individual or panels of nursing home patients.

Medicare reimbursement would also encourage nursing homes to employ GNPs directly. Since nursing homes may now salary physicians and bill Medicare Part B for the medical care they provide, extending Part B payments to GNPs would genuinely and appropriately encourage GNP employment in nursing homes.

An ongoing concern of nursing homes is quality of medical coverage. Despite a predicted physician surplus, physicians continue to avoid nursing home visits. Nursing home administrators feel powerless to alter physician behavior, and frequently the medical directors' primary function is that of policing other physicians' quality of care. Nurses in nursing homes lament their inability to institute appropriate and timely care due to the inaccessability of physicians. Reimbursement of GNPs for some medical services would allow nursing homes to negotiate practice arrangements with physicians and GNPs which would improve the quality of medical coverage. For example, in negotiating medical privileges, the home could request that a GNP make nursing home visits on a prearranged and regularly scheduled basis. Nursing homes could encourage patients to select physicians who have collaborative arrangements with GNPs, emphasizing increased access to care that the GNP provides. When the patient has no primary provider, the nursing home preferentially could assign primary care to an MD/GNP team over a physician practicing without GNP collaboration or the home could employ the GNP, develop collaborative physician arrangements, and bill directly for GNP reimbursable services.

Permitting GNPs to assume some duties of the medical director would further encourage employment of GNPs in nursing homes. Under HCFA Conditions of Participation, the medical director in a nursing home reviews patient policies and incident reports, establishes medical policies and procedures, and participates in selected committees. Given that many mandated functions of the medical director are well within the scope of practice by a GNP, the position could be redefined to allow GNPs to fulfill some directorial functions. Homes could be required to establish consultant medical committees to develop policies regarding specialized needs, for example infection control.

The substitution of a GNP to serve certain functions of the medical director would allow some current spending to be redirected to cover a portion of the GNPs salary. Despite the salary differential between GNPs and physicians, it is unlikely that diverted funds would cover a significant share of the GNPs total salary given the part-time nature of most medical director positions. Nevertheless, having this option may induce some nursing homes to employ GNPs. The major disadvantage in suggesting that the position of medical director be waived or reconstituted is the further erosion of an already limited physician presence in nursing homes.

Increasing Medicare reimbursements for nursing homes who care for large numbers of patients with high acuity and who employ GNPs is a third option for encourageing GNP employment in nursing homes. Some nursing home patients are sufficiently ill, as are patients in specialty units of a hospital, to require the presence and supervision of a nurse specialist. PPS is increasing the population needing highly skilled post-hospital care so there will be more nursing homes serving a larger number of these patients. Many Medicaid case mix nursing home reimbursement systems already provide incentives for care of sicker patients, and in some instances have differentially reimbursed for care by GNPs. In Ohio, for example, two participating RWJF TNHPs have demonstrated that the increased care given by GNPs warrants a higher level of Medicaid reimbursement.

Designation of a second level of care for Medicare, the "super SNF," could also be a step toward a casemix payment system under Medicare. There is an important distinction, however. Unlike some Medicaid casemix systems which pay on the basis of patients care needs regardless of the home's resources to fulfill those needs, higher payments would go only to facilities employing the extra resources and fulfilling the other standards of a super SNF. Facilities not satisfying these standards would not qualify for higher payment even when they had patients who met super SNF criteria.

Under current reimbursement policies, designation of a separate level of care would likely mean that qualifying facilities would face a separate and potentially higher ceiling on their reimbursable costs. This would represent an incentive to become a super SNF only for those high cost facilities already above their ceiling. If Medicare wishes to encourage more strongly the development of super SNFs, it must modify its payment system to provide explicit profits. One of Medicare's continued shortcomings in gaining access to nursing homes for its beneficiaries is a failure to recognize that the program's leverage is limited. As a small purchaser of care, nursing homes can ignore Medicare of its requirements are too demanding and the reimbursement not attractive enough.

The impact of increased involvement of GNPs in nursing homes needs to be considered from the perspective of the patient, the practitioner, and the home. For the patient, substitution of nursing home care for hospital care can be of some concern. The trauma of an institutional transfer may be avoided, but will outcomes be the same? Sensitivity by GNPs to the home's capabilities compared to the hospital will need to be weighed carefully when making decisions about treatment.

In order to maximize the potential cost savings which accrue from providing timely treatment that substitutes for more expensive services, GNPs must have the flexibility and incentive to monitor patients closely and intervene whenever necessary. Current rules restricting Medicare payments to medical emergencies between specified intervals which undermine timely treatment should be broadened. If payment is repeatedly retrospectively denied, GNPs will be deterred as are their physician colleagues from providing preventive care.

A possibility, which will likely be discussed, is some form of capitated or package reimbursement for mandated medical services to be provided by salaried physicians and/or GNPs. This may be of particular interest in light of ongoing attempts to establish physician DRGs. Physician DRGs currently are envisioned as fixed case payment per hospital admission with the size of the payment determined by the patient's DRG. Under physician DRGs "all services performed by physicians and normally billed as Part B services would be combined into a single bill and a single payment." This would be similar to current packaging or bundling of services which applies to obstetricians for an episode of pregnancy.[32]

For nursing home patients, packaged payment would likely be for a unit of time, say a month. The extreme variability of nursing home lengths of stay and resources needed during a given stay preclude per case payments. Capitated payment would provide flexibility to medical care providers to administer care as needed while establishing control over costs for Medicare. Two significant concerns outweigh these advantages. First, a single physician or GNP or group practice would require a sufficient number of nursing home patients to legitimately offset the risk of having a very costly patient. The Massachusetts Waiver Program suggests that this may be problematical for a significant number of providers. The second concern is the presence of some mechanism associated with capitated or package payments which would guard against underprovision. In this instance, such a coutervailing force is not present and therefore would need to be created. Nursing home patients, being very old and very sick whose families are resigned to poor prognoses, are extremely vulnerable. It would be essential to create an independent entity to monitor the adequacy and quality of care delivery. Even then, the efficacy of this independent regulator would be open to question and the programmatic savings generated from packaged payments versus a fee for service may not be sufficient to justify the risk.

Nursing homes may welcome GNPs who provide improved care. However, the nursing homes may be less sanguine about keeping sicker patients who would otherwise be transferred to hospitals if adequate compensation for the additional resources such care requires is not forthcoming. Nursing homes profit from hospitalized patients. Medicaid programs and private patients often pay to reserve nursing home beds while patients are hospitalized. Inducing the nursing home to care for sicker patients likely will require at least some additional reimbursement, or better yet, the earning of additional profit. This will not be easy to achieve because the principal payers of nursing home costs are Medicaid programs and private patients, while the beneficiary of reduced hospital costs is Medicare.

Ironically, though several state Medicaid programs have changed their reimbursement systems to vary payment according to severity of patient's condition (i.e., case mix reimbursement systems) financial gains from these systems remain unclear. These systems encourage and accommodate the care of sicker patients in nursing homes. However, the systems do not always respond immediately to a patient's worsening condition. To avoid excessive assessment costs and to avoid creating rewards for a more dependent or sicker patient, systems often adjust to patient classifications and thereby pay at specified intervals. Exceptions are made, but some permit unscheduled reclassifications only after a hospitalization. Overall, it would be expected that the cooperation of the nursing home in accommodating the expanded GNP role would be sufficient to generate net cost savings. Fragmentation among payment sources will, however, make it more difficult to accommodate the expanded role of the GNP, in spite of the generated savings in costs.

Whether or not the GNP is responsible primarily to the patient or the nursing home is also complicated. As an agent of the patient (i.e., either as an employee of an HMO or in collaborative practice with a physician), the GNP makes clinical decisions unconstrained by nursing home needs or concerns. Cost savings resulting from care by the GNP are easily demonstrable, as in the Massachusetts Waiver Program. Nevertheless, the presence of the GNP in the nursing home is still episodic. The GNP remains an outsider to the staff and patient contacts are limited. Moreover, in such arrangements GNPs are subject to the same demand for efficiency and productivity which prevail for physicians; needless to say this may have the opposite of the desired effect, namely further limitations to patient contact.

On the other hand, when GNPs are based in the facility, their services are available to staff and patients on a continuing basis and they can more readily provide both physician-substitute and nursing services. Daily contact with patients enhances GNP's role in prevention of disease and timely response to symptoms. GNPs more readily gain the staff's trust and augment supervisory, inservice, and quality assurance activities. Nevertheless, there are disadvantages to facility-based employment of GNPs. Effectiveness may be limited by diffusing the practitioner's efforts over a large number of tasks, some of which are not specific or appropriate to the GNP role.[33] In addition, there is a potential source of conflict between the GNP and nursing home when the GNP selects a treatment plan which is not necessarily the most cost-effective option. Mechanisms need to be in place which assure that GNPs have sufficient independence and control of practice to make appropriate decisions about treatment, irrespective of cost.

Market forces should determine the provider model (i.e., physician alone, GNP/physician collaborative practice, or nursing home employment of GNPs), that best suits regional and individual nursing home and patient needs. In regions where GNPs are unavailable, physicians would continue to provide the bulk of care to nursing home residents. On the other hand, in areas where GNPs are available in sufficient numbers, nursing homes could choose to contract with physicians and GNPs in ways that best meet the care needs of patients.

Advocacy of payment to cover participation by GNPs in nursing homes may seem like heresy in an era of cost containment. However, if such expenditures result in Medicare Part A and B cost savings, not spending such money could be characterized as extreme myopia.

REFERENCES

1. U.S. Department of Health and Human Services (DHHS), Press Release, June 23, 1987.
2. US Senate Special Committee on Aging. *Nursing home care:* (Serial 99–5) *The Unfinished agenda.* Washington, DC: U.S. Government Printing Office; 1986.
3. Doty P, Liu K, Weiner J. Special report: An overview of long-term care. *Health Care Financing Rev* 1985; 6:69–78.
4. U.S. General Accounting Office. *Medicaid and nursing home care: Cost increases and the need for services are creating problems for the states and the elderly* (Report No. GAO/IPE-84-1). Washington, DC: U.S. Government Printing Office; 1983.
5. Loeser W, Dickstein E, Schiavoke L. Medicare coverage in nursing homes— a broken promise. *N Eng J Med* 1981; 304:353–5.
6. U.S. DHHS, op. cit.
7. Gruenberg L, Willemain T. Hospital discharge queue in Massachusetts. *Med Care* 1982; 20:20–27.
8. Lewis M, Leake B, Leal-Sotelo M, Clark V. The initial effects of the prospective payment system on nursing home patients. *Am. J. Public Health* 1987; 77:819–821.
9. Mitchell J. *Physician DRGs: What do they look like and how do they work.* Chestnut Hill MA: Health Economics Research, Inc., 1985.
10. U.S. DHHS, Federal Regulations 1976; 76:41.
11. Aiken L. Nursing priorities for the 1980s: Hospitals and nursing homes. *Am J Nurs* 1981; 81:324–30.
12. Mitchell J, Hewes H. *Medicare access to physician services in nursing homes.* Final report for Health Care Financing Administration (Grant No. 95-P-97885/1). Boston, MA: Center for Health Research; 1982.
13. Domoto K, Ben R, Wei J, Pass T, Komoroff A. Yield of routine annual laboratory screening in the institutionalized elderly. *Am J Public Health* 1985; 75:243–5.
14. Lamy P. *Prescribing for the elderly.* Littleton MA: PSG Publishing; 1981.
15. Kramer M. Trends of institutionalization and prevalence of mental disorders in nursing homes. In: M. Harper and B. Lebowitz, eds. *Mental Illness in Nursing Homes: Agenda for Research* (DHHS Publication No. (ADM) 86-1459). Washington, DC: National Institute of Mental Health; 1986.

16. U.S. Congress Office of Technology Assessment. *Nurse practitioners, physician assistants, and certified nurse-midwives: A policy analysis* (Health Technology Case Study 37, OTA-HCS-37). Washington, DC: U.S. Government Printing Office; 1986.
17. Mezey M, McGivern D, eds. *Nurses, nurse practitioners: The evolution of primary care.* Boston, MA: Little, Brown and Co; 1986.
18. Freund C. Nurse practitioners in primary care. In: Mezey M, McGivern D, eds. *Nurses, nurse practitioners: The evolution of primary care.* Boston, MA: Little, Brown and Co; 1986.
19. U.S. Congress Office of Technology Assessment, op cit, p. 41.
20. Master R, Feltin M, Jainchill J, Mark R, Kavish W, Rabkin M, Turner B, Bachrach S, Lennox S. A Continuance of Care for the Innercity: assessment of its benefits for Boston's elderly and high-risk populations. *N Engl J Med* 1980; 302:1434–40.
21. Mezey M, Lynaugh J, Aiken L. The Robert Wood Johnson Foundation teaching nursing home. In: E Schreider, ed. *The teaching nursing home: A new approach to geriatric education, research, and medical care.* New York: Raven Press; 1985.
22. Ebersole P. Gerontological nurse practitioners past and present. *Geriatr Nurs* 1985; 6:219–22.
23. Wieland D, Rubenstein L, Ouslander J, Martin S. Organizing an academic nursing home. *J Am Med Assoc* 1986; 255:2622–27.
24. Department of Welfare *Case-managed medical care for nursing home patients.* (Massachusetts 1115 waiver program). Boston, MA: Author; 1987.
25. Group Health of Puget Sound, personal communication.
26. Kaiser Permanente, Portland, Oregon, personal communication, 1987.
27. Henderson M. A GNP in a retirement community. *Geriatr Nurs* 1984; 5:109–12.
28. Kummerer-Butler J. Life care community practice. In: Mezey M, McGivern D, eds. *Nurses, nurse practitioners: The evolution of primary care.* Boston, MA: Little, Brown and Co.; 1986.
29. U.S. Congress Office of Technology Assessment, op. cit. p. 9.
30. op. cit. p. 9.
31. S.2920 The Advanced Nursing Services in Nursing Homes Act, 1986.
32. Mitchell J, Hewes H, op. cit.
33. Kane R, Garrard J, Buchanan J, Arnold S, Kane R, McDermott S. The geriatric nurse practitioner as a nursing home employee: Conceptual and methodological issues in assessing quality of care and cost effectiveness. In: Mezey M, Lynaugh J, eds. *Nursing homes and nursing care: Lessons from the teaching nursing homes.* New York: Springer Publishing Co., 1988.

6

Four Examples of Academic Involvement in Nursing Home Care

CASE A
Johns Hopkins University: An Academic Health Center and Long-Term Care

Robert Heyssel

Nursing homes have received short shrift from academic health centers. Negotiations about patient transfers are generally the only professional contact that an academic health center has with a nursing home. Few, if any, medical schools use nursing homes as a clinical teaching site—the reason may be that academic medicine has little interest in teaching geriatrics or in gerontological research. Even university schools of nursing distance themselves from nursing homes—although the very name implies that nursing is central to what the homes do.

This long-standing professional disinterest and disengagement has its roots in the preoccupation of medicine with acute illness and in the perception within the nursing profession that nursing home work is not the career of choice. Finally, there is the bottom line: reimbursement programs for nursing homes do not provide for the traditional piggybacking of research and educational costs that have so amply supported medical education and research in our teaching hospitals.

Academic health centers will have to change their attitudes about nursing homes because of demographic and economic pressures. These include a rapidly aging population, declining occupancy rates in acute care hospitals, and a health care delivery system that is drastically being changed by Medicare Prospective Payment. The emerging vertically integrated systems of health care equally are important.

We are fast moving away from the old concept of the hospital as an independent setting for acute care which relies on private physicians and group practices to fill patient beds. The hospital of today, particularly the urban hospital with its ambulatory care clinics, is rapidly becoming one of the links in a closely-knit chain of medical care. The links are many: ambulatory care, alternative delivery systems such as HMOs and PPOs, community-based urgent care centers, home health care, and nursing home care. These are often coupled with fitness centers and preventive programs operated by the hospital. It is likely that, in the next decade, many of our major hospitals and academic health centers will be establishing similar systems on a local and regional basis. Despite Paul Ellwood's prediction, I do not think that a dozen "Super-med" systems will emerge on a national basis. I do think that, depending on the size of the urban center, local and regional hospital/academic health center affiliations will eventually give rise to two or three regional vertically-integrated systems of care. It is these regional systems that will be competing with one another.

None too soon, medical schools have come to realize the importance of geriatric medicine. Even if our health care system were not being reshaped by payment changes, competition, cost containment, and physician surplus, the reality of a rapidly growing elderly population would of itself create interest in geriatric medicine. Medical schools are beginning to rethink their curriculum and consider whether medical students would benefit from clinical instruction in nursing homes.

Apart from teaching and research, the benefits to the patients themselves argue in favor of extended formal linkages between the nursing home and the acute hospital. The hospital and the nursing home could work together in supervising the care of patients transferred from one facility to another. This would help to decrease the risk of hospitalization and facilitate patient transfers when appropriate. This type of relationship could "medicalize" the nursing home and create costs that are socially and medically unnecessary. That seems unlikely, given the payment system and the increasing competition within the health care delivery system.

I have referred to vertically-integrated systems of care but will now provide an example of how such a system developed at Johns Hopkins. First, a bit of history about how all the pieces came together.

Long before we began to develop our system of care, Johns Hopkins had a relationship with Baltimore City Hospitals which included the acute hospital and Mason F. Lord Chronic Care Facility. The chronic care facility consisted of a 160-bed skilled nursing facility and a chronic hospital, with 60-medical-surgical beds. The Gerontological Research Center of the National Institute of Aging is also located on the grounds of the Baltimore City Hospitals.

So many resources so close at hand—a nursing home, a chronic care facility, and a major research center on aging—made the care of the aged and the dependent at least a peripheral interest at Johns Hopkins, although the number of medical school faculty with an active interest in geriatrics was very small. The fact was that faculty interest in the care of the aged had more to do with geography, convenient facilities, and Johns Hopkins' involvement with Baltimore City Hospitals than with any deliberate or academic programming by Johns Hopkins itself.

In 1984, Johns Hopkins assumed the management of Baltimore City Hospitals. The following year, we acquired Baltimore City Hospitals (acute and chronic divisions) from the City of Baltimore. Subsequently, Baltimore City Hospitals was renamed the Francis Scott Key Medical Center. During the same period, we acquired two additional hospitals. These four hospitals and an HMO, developed and owned by Johns Hopkins, are operated by a new corporate entity: The Johns Hopkins Health System, a not-for-profit holding company.

Our HMO, called the Johns Hopkins Health Plan, covers the Baltimore metropolitan region. A network of seven hospitals in addition to the four hospitals in the Johns Hopkins Health System, participates in our HMO-PPO activities. This hospital network gives our HMO patients the widest possible coverage in terms of gerographical location and medical care. Another important advantage of our vertically-integrated system of care is cost-effective management strategies such as joint purchasing programs and a laboratory corporation which service the hospitals and the Health Plan. These cost-efficient measures result in savings to the individual institutions and therefore to the patients as well.

One of the links in the Johns Hopkins Health System is the Mason F. Lord Home at Francis Scott Key Medical Center. We plan to replace the present building which is outmoded with a new modern nursing home facility. The newly accreditied Johns Hopkins School of Nursing will use the new Mason F. Lord Home as a setting for nursing education, research, and practice. The Home will be a major education site for the Johns Hopkins School of Medicine at both the undergraduate and graduate levels. We expect that the Home will be a principal site for research programs under the aegis of the National Institute of Aging.

We expect that in the near future most of the patients in the Mason F. Lord Home will come from the Johns Hopkins Health System. The problem is that we have 56,000 to 60,000 discharges a year and the Home's 240 beds will not be able to accommodate all those who will require nursing home care. We will undoubtedly make arrangements with other nursing homes over time but through affiliation rather than ownership capacity.

The Johns Hopkins Health System is already preparing to cope with the health care needs of the growing population of AIDS patients (which is doubling every six months.) Approximately 40% of those with AIDS and AIDS-related complex are going to require nursing home care at some point. At present, only two nursing homes in the Baltimore area will accept AIDS patients. Representatives of the Johns Hopkins Health System and an investor-owned nursing home chain are discussing the joint development and operation of a nursing home specifically for AIDS patients. The facility would also have an adjunct day-care hospital and home health services.

As vertically-integrated systems of care begin to develop around academic health centers and large hospitals, especially teaching hospitals, interest in nursing homes and nursing home operations is certain to rise. This interest will be the catalyst for more intensive programs in teaching and research within the nursing home environment. Such programs have been a long time coming and they are desperately needed. It is only through such programs that the quality of care for the dependent elderly will improve, that the most appropriate care will be offered at the best site, that the risk of unnecessary hospitalization will be reduced, and that unwarranted terminal care in the hospital will be avoided.

CASE B
Oregon Health Science University School of Nursing and the Benedictine Nursing Center: The University Perspective

Carol Lindeman

The graying of America has made nursing homes one of the nation's hottest health care issues. Nursing homes are currently the fastest growing sector of health care facilities in the Unites States, and this unprecedented growth creates concern about standards of care and the availability of qualified professional caregivers. The concern is a realistic one, for nursing homes compete for a limited pool of nurses, physicians, and others trained in the special care requirements of the institutionalized elderly.

The challenge presented by the Teaching Nursing Home program is significant for nursing and for society. In the abstract, the challenge was: Can new partnerships be created within the health care and educational sectors that will address the social problems caused by a rapidly growing elderly population, an inadequate long-term care delivery system, and a limited supply of health professionals interested in gerontology? On a more concrete level, the challenge was: Can a university school of nursing and a nursing home form a partnership to improve the quality of care in the nursing home, enhance the quality and quantity of educational experiences in long-term care, and interest future practitioners in gerontology careers?

THE TEACHING NURSING HOME PROGRAM: THE AGGREGATE EXPERIENCE

The Robert Wood Johnson Teaching Nursing Home Program concluded in 1987. At that time, the eleven university schools of nursing and nursing homes which affiliated for the program informally reported on the advantages and disadvantages associated with the implementation of the Teaching Nursing Home Program.

The first and most positive outcome was that a majority of the sites indicated they most definitely would submit a grant application if they had to do it over again. Some sites even reported that they were developing additional affiliations as a result of the Teaching Nursing Home experience.

The advantages most frequently cited were faculty role development, improved image of university school of nursing, research development and utilization, and advanced practice roles. The disadvantages most frequently cited were issues related to conflicts between the academic and clinical settings, and organizational complexity. These benefits and drawbacks are summarized briefly in the following sections.

ADVANTAGES OF THE TEACHING NURSING HOME PROGRAM

Teaching–Learning Process

The overall excellence of the Teaching Nursing Home as a clinical site was mentioned most frequently. Respondents reported that the program gave undergraduate and graduate students learning opportunities and hands-on experiences in caring for the elderly. Because a student could care for the same client over a prolonged period there was continuity in learning. In turn, the student received positive feedback from the residents. Graduate students were able to learn management skills in addition to direct patient care. Because faculty members had greater control over the clinical experience, they were able to prepare students and guide their experience more effectively. The best measure of the effectiveness of the Teaching Nursing Home is the desire of students to enter nursing home practice after graduation.

Faculty Role Development

The Teaching Nursing Home facilitated faculty development in several significant areas. Faculty members who are sensitive to the needs of the elderly developed a curriculum that reflected the real world of practice. As their understanding and accountability for the quality of care in the clinical setting increased, so did their interest and expertise in legislative issues related to long-term care. New and expanded knowledge in a wide range of gerontological issues led to increased faculty publications. On the interpersonal level, faculty were able to deal with students' criticisms of the system from the perspective of staff. On the personal level, faculty enjoyed the satisfaction of caring for the elderly and showed greater creativity in their academic and clinical teaching.

Image of University School of Nursing

The Teaching Nursing Home Program affiliations created a much more favorable public image of the schools of nursing. As faculty and students became involved in community programs for the elderly, the community began to see the schools as genuinely concerned with social issues. The national visibility given to faculty and their schools helped to attract new faculty in rehabilitation, geropsychiatry, and gerontological nursing and at the same time increase enrollment in other educational programs. Finally, the Program was the impetus for establishing a national interdisciplinary gerontologic/geriatric network and a nursing network in the clinical arena.

Research Development and Utilization

The Teaching Nursing Home Program provided ready access to appropriate study populations for testing new nursing interventions and for generating and testing nursing theory. Nurses could apply academic concepts in the clinical setting, thereby generating new knowledge about the delivery of care to the elderly. Faculty and students were actively involved in restructuring the system of care delivery as part of the quality assurance program. Increased numbers of collaborative research projects, professional presentations, and publications related to the Program have sparked the interest of other faculty in long-term care.

Advanced Practice Roles

The Teaching Nurse Program was an opportunity to demonstrate a nursing model for long-term care. This initiative enabled faculty to serve as clinical role models for staff and students. It also demonstrated the potential of master's prepared clinical nurse specialists to improve the quality of patient care in nursing homes.

DISADVANTAGES OF THE TEACHING NURSING HOME PROGRAM

Academic Setting Issues

University schools of nursing find that marginal financing and a limited pool of academic nurses qualified for faculty positions tend to stretch their faculty thinly. This situation of overextended, overtaxed faculty can help to explain why the Teaching Nursing Home Program may not have received full faculty support. It must be remembered that the Program began In 1981 when resources for higher education were beginning their decline, which made the Program a competitor for scarce dollars. Many faculty, who did not understand the teaching nursing home concept, perceived the affiliation with a nursing home as conflicting with university facilities or with existing clinical affiliations. Furthermore, the off-campus site had no immediate visibility. In general, senior faculty tended not to be interested in the program while doctorally-prepared assistant professors were pressured by the pull between service needs and scholarly activities.

Clinical Setting Issues

As was the case in the academic setting, there was little understanding of the teaching nursing home concept in the clinical setting, particularly since nursing homes are generally isolated from the mainstream of nursing. Staffing was a constant problem. Personnel were not well prepared for their roles, and few role models were available. A high turnover in administrative personnel and a reluctance to share decision making further complicated matters. Reimbursement issues impeded efforts to initiate changes, and reimubrsement problems became the nursing home rationale for maintaining the status quo. Moreover, few in the clinical setting understood the importance of nursing research.

Organizational Issues

The university schools of nursing and the nursing homes often had difficulties in appreciating the external and internal pressures faced by the other. Finances, values, beliefs, and goals were among the major areas of misunderstanding. Developing the school/home relationship required extensive time and energy. The Teaching Nursing Home affiliation was essentially an agreement among people difficult to move to a full-fledged organizational accomplishment. The schools and the homes found that establishing mutual trust and lines of communication was difficult and time-consuming.

OHSU AND THE TEACHING NURSING HOME PROGRAM

The Oregon Health Science University (OHSU) School of Nursing was eager to participate in The Robert Wood Johnson Teaching Nursing Home Program for two major reasons. First, the faculty of the School of Nursing had decided to limit the number of agencies used for clinical experience and to develop collaborative models with those agencies. Such arrangements were already underway with the University Hospital and with the Veterans Administration Medical Center. The Teaching Nursing Home thus aligned itself with that goal. Second, the faculty was committed to gerontological nursing, and the School had initiated clinical teaching facilities and didactic courses at undergraduate and graduate levels. In the 1970s, the faculty had developed a proposal for the School to purchase a nursing home. The Teaching Nursing Home Program was an opportunity that matched existing interst and goals.

Our previous experiences had shown that any affiliation, in order to be successful, had to begin with an agency which possesses a strong sense of identity, strength, and quality. OHSU School of Nursing therefore proposed an affiliation with a nursing home recognized for its quality and values—the Benedictine Nursing Center.

PARTNERS IN THE TEACHING NURSING HOME PROGRAM

OHSU School of Nursing: An Overview

The OHSU School of Nursing has a reputation for sound and innovative programs of education and research. Its highly qualified professoriate includes 40 doctorally-prepared faculty members. For the last three years, the School has received Biomedical Research Support Grant funds in recognition of its research productivity. During the same period, faculty members have presented over 390 papers at local, state, regional national and international meetings. During the last five years, faculty members have published approximately 345 scholarly papers. Much of the research funding and many of the faculty presentations relate to gerontology and long-term care.

The nursing faculty role demands accountability for excellence in practice and teaching, active participation in research, publication, and community service. To support faculty in these activities and to facilitate joint projects with clinical agencies, the School has a clinical practice arrangement with the University Hospital; an Office of Nursing Research Development and Utilization that is jointly funded by the School and hospital and includes a director, statistician, three nurse researchers, and research assistants; and a Joint Venture Project with the Portland Veterans Administration Medical Center.

The School has an undergraduate program for generic and registered nurses in Portland (300 students) and in La Grande (60 students), a master's program in Portland (100 students) and in Medford (40 students), and a doctoral program in Portland (30 students). Nursing alumni hold leadership positions as directors of nursing service, clinical nurse specialists, nurse practitioners, and educators. The School's continuing education programs includes many courses directly related to the care of the elderly.

Care of the elderly is the concern of all departments of the School of Nursing. The graduate program in gerontological nursing, funded by the Division of Nursing, has increased resources for teaching, research, and practice related to the elderly. Undergraduate students receive three credit hours of theory and five of practice related to the elderly. Graduate students may pursue an interest in gerontology either through a clinical major in medical-surgical, mental health, or gerontological nursing, or through an administration major with emphasis on health care delivery to the elderly. Gerontological nursing majors earn 17 credit hours through classroom and clinical experience that integrates research, theory, and practice.

The Benedictine Nursing Center: An Overview

The Benedictine Nursing Center (BNC) is widely known and respected for providing high quality professional services for the elderly, the chronically ill, the disabled, and the dying in a supportive, loving environment that meets human needs through a holistic approach. The Center's goals include maintaining a strong financial base in order to carry out its mission, serving as a role model by facilitating and promoting progressive approaches in the field of long-term care, and advocating for the elderly and chronically ill in matters of public policy and health care delivery.

The Benedictine Nursing Center is located in the rural area of Mount Angel, Oregon. Founded in 1955 by local residents as a 20-bed home for the aged, the Center currently serves local communities within a twenty-mile radius. The Center, which is under the direction of a volunteer board, has 127 residents and 75 home health care patients at various levels of care. The Center provides some support to those on its waiting list. A major concern of the Center is that those who are admitted often cannot find community-based alternatives to an extended nursing home stay. The BNC director and board perceived the Teaching Nursing Home innovation as critical to the issues of long-term care and the ways of delivering that care to the elderly. They welcomed the challenge presented by the Robert Wood Johnson Foundation Teaching Nursing Home Program.

The Center's staff is multidisciplinary. The nursing home team consists of an associate administrator who is a nurse, a director and an assistant director of nursing service, thirty-five nurses, two clinical specialists, a social worker, three therapists, an activities coordinator, and a dietician. The medical director, a local physician, serves as consultant to the administrator and staff. Each resident in the facility also has a personal attending physician. The Center has transfer agreements with Silverton and Salem Hospitals. Other hospitals are resources for referral and care. Dental and podiatry services are provided on an individual basis. A gerontolgial psychiatrist consults regularly with the team. Shared decision making and open communication among the team are encouraged.

The Center is the clinical site for students from Chemeketa Community College, occupational and physical therapy students from Pacific University, and through the Teaching Nursing Home Program, students from OHSU School of Nursing; and a training site for nursing aides. The Center also sponsors biannual conferences concerning issues related to the elderly. Additional programs, open to others, are provided for BNC employees. Staff are given financial assistance to attend other workshops.

The Center periodically reviews its progress and evaluates its programs through a facility-wide question and answer program.

ADVANTAGES AND DISADVANTAGES FROM THE PERSPECTIVE OF A DEAN

Initially, we were sure we knew what a Teaching Nursing Home Program was. We very quickly discovered that we had much to learn. The goals were clear: to improve educational experiences for nursing students and to improve the quality of care for nursing home residents. Once the program got underway, however, we began to wonder how we were going to achieve those goals within the context of a collaborative model. Each year became a time of discovery and learning, and each year moved us closer to our goals. In the end, it was our mutual commitment to those goals and a willingness to trust one another that resulted in our success. The reality was far different from what we pictured in 1981 when we wrote the grant application.

From the OHSU perspective, the Teaching Nursing Home Program had two primary advantages. First, faculty growth and development were enhanced by the rich learning environment of the Benedictine Nursing Center. Second, student growth and development were improved by clinical experiences in a long-term care facility where quality care is the norm. The difficulties we encountered were those associated with any truly innovative endeavor. We have not yet developed schoolwide ownership of the program since the affiliation too often is perceived as a program of the Community Health Care Systems Department where the grant was housed. The only major disadvantage of the Program had to do with geography. Life would have been much simpler had the Benedictine Nursing Center been housed on the OHSU campus rather than 40 miles away, or so we thought.

In general, the School's experience in the Teaching Nursing Home program has been overwhelmingly positive. We are committed to an ongoing affiliation and, to date, have agreed to continue joint funding for two clinical specialists and to operate an Institute for Research and Education in Long-term Care. The affiliation has enabled the School to obtain new training monies. We anticipate that the affiliation will also help us attract new research funds as current pilot studies move forward.

SUMMARY

An affiliation between a university-based school of nursing and a nursing home strengthens nursing home care; interests health professionals in long-term care; increases opportunities for teaching, for research, and for the dissemination of knowledge regarding long-term care; and enhances the vitality and visibility of a school of nursing. Accomplishing these goals is arduous and time-consuming and financial assistance is essential.

University schools of nursing have struggled to define and retain what is essential to the discipline of nursing in a shark-filled academic environment. The pressure of the affiliation strains these nursing essentials and can stir up past feelings of mistrust. Neither partner in the affiliation should have to surrender values or beliefs, its essential parts.

The affiliation is more than two organizations agreeing to terms set down in a protocol. Above all, the affiliation is a human process, a melding of values, beliefs, dreams, and constraints. It is a relationship that reminds me of a quote from May Sarton: "No partner in a love relationship should feel that he has to give up an essential part of himself to make it viable."

CASE C
Creighton University and Madonna Professional Care Center/Mercy Care Center: One Dean's Experience

Sheila Ryan

The strategy of the Creighton University Teaching Nursing Home Program (TNHP) was simple: to share resources, faculty/staff, ideas, data, and move from a competitive to a cooperative reality. Our TNH accomplishments are numerous. Gerontological nurse clinician faculty worked with nursing home staff to remedy clinical problems which plague nursing home patients (i.e., falls, infections, decubiti, incontinence, spitting, name calling, depression, sensory losses, social resources, and dependency). We believe we were effective in decreasing emergency room visits, hospital stays, and even nursing home lengths of stay.

The low ratio of professional nursing staff in nursing homes was an initial shock to faculty. During the project's first month, one faculty member came in and said. "You won't believe the staffing! We need to do something about it!" The importance of demonstrating quality of care was underscored, and faculty were heavily invested in documenting quality of care and the effectiveness of standards. Faculty began classes for ANA certification in gerontological nursing for staff nurses in nursing homes. They chose clinical problems which concerned nursing home patients and staff as research topics. For example, the nationally-funded study to develop an instrument, the Braden Scale, to predict the risk of skin breakdown[1] holds great promise for nursing home residents. Faculty assisted in developing media productions to alert consumers regarding issues of quality of care for the elderly in general and for nursing home patients in particular. They initiated radio spots and health tips for the elderly, for example, on the effect of hypothermia during very cold winters in Nebraska; they prepared video tapes on Alzheimer's disease to support family caregivers, and on discharge planning as a teaching tool for nursing homes. Finally, faculty delivered lectures and served as consultants on issues of long-term care to legislatures, health associations, and regional health departments throughout the state. One faculty member who testified at legislative hearings temporarily influenced hospital based nursing home rates by showing that the acuity levels of many skilled nursing residents were higher than in some hospital-based patients. Others offered testimony on living wills, wrote rules and regulations for nursing home staff, and prepared a bill on case management for the elderly.

Much of the TNH success lies in the changed attitudes and experiences of students. By exposing undergraduate and graduate students to more gerontological content, to interdisciplinary experiences with physicians, dentists, pharmacists and social workers, and by offering students opportunities to co-lead patient and staff groups, students now appreciate the complexity of nursing home practice. When one student entered the intensive care rotation of our affiliated hospital, she was heard to comment "Oh! It's the nursing home with respirators!"

The Teaching Nursing Home Program final report will be enriched by slightly different examples from the other 10 TNH sites across the country. However, I would like to add my own descriptive colors and stories to this growing collage . . . to describe how the Teaching Nursing Home Program became a driving force behind a community linked model of faculty practice with a special focus on the elderly (see Figure 6.1).

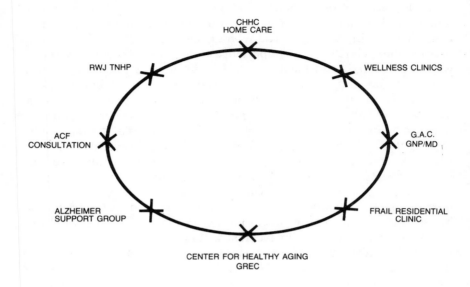

Figure 6.1 Community Linked Model of Faculty Practice

The TNHP made it easier for faculty to become fully involved in another project whereby the school of nursing became a fully approved and certified home health care agency. This home care agency now delivers approximately 350 visits a month; of those visits, 70 to 80% are made by students and faculty.[2] The following example helps to illustrate how faculty and students working together on clinical problems created both a better answer to the problems and an ideal learning experience. A few years ago, quality assurance was a topic that students learned in a 2-hour lecture from a faculty expert. To meet Medicare requirements as a home health care agency, however, we needed to audit randomly 10% of the charts on a quarterly basis. Faculty immediately asked, "When are we going to have time to do this?" "Why do *you* need to do it?" was the reply. A group of faculty and students analyzed, revised and improved the criteria, and developed a routine of monthly 25% random chart audits conducted by students. As a result, the State Health Department commended the agency, saying it was the best quality assurance system in the state. It led to no loss and, temporarily, to an increase in reimbursement.

Recognizing our interest and accomplishments in clinical care, the Eastern Nebraska Office on Aging approached the school and asked if we would submit a competitive bid for 30 nursing home clinics at nutritional sites for the elderly. We were discouraged by several colleagues from pursuing this contract because it appeared to compete with the local Visiting Nurse Association (VNA). But we won the bid over six other proposals because we presented a quality proposal at a lower cost. As a result of this contract, we conducted intensive assessments on functionally independent elderly in our community. The proposal was cost effective because it used faculty, students, and volunteer nurses from the community to conduct the assessments. Two faculty reported on the data collected on approximately 700 independent elderly to multiple audiences.[3] After one year, the VNA and Creighton nursing faculty shared the contract; we learned that working together could enhance all of our resources and still meet different institutional missions.

One of our favorite projects was a demonstration project funded by our Office on New Initiatives at Creighton. This was an independent nursing clinic serving 170 frail elderly (average age, 83) and set in a residential home.[4] Through trial and error, we learned that clients would rarely make appointments for health promotion visits when we used a care system modeled on a physician's office. Rather, health promotion services were best delivered where the residents lived: in the cafeteria, card game rooms, classrooms, and in residents' apartments. We also learned that the elderly would not pay for health promotion services, no matter what payment options were offered (i.e., fee for service, fee for time spent, or preferred provider option). Originally, we envisioned that a modified nursing PPO would be an ideal payment option. For the price of a monthly hair permanent, even with only 60% of residents participating we could cover the program's cost. Elderly residents, however, accustomed to using their Medicare card to cover most health services, were unwilling to subscribe. But their adult working children *were* willing to pay for this service. They wanted a professional to advise them when a parent fell ill or their mental status changed. As the primary care providers in these situations, faculty clinicians could advise family members when the situation warranted a physician's appointment or possibly an emergency room visit. This information helped families avoid unnecessary hours, expense, and anxiety seeking a professional opinion. Though the initial program goals were not to deliver advice regarding the need for physician and emergency services, we quickly learned to market this aspect of the program in order to pay for the health promotion. The success of this project, including its potential to be self-funding, influenced the facility administrator to hire a full-time professional nurse, and faculty now act in an advisory capacity.

Most important was the development of an all university interdisciplinary Committee on Aging, currently chaired by a school of nursing faculty member. This committee facilitated the collaborative practice of a geriatric nurse practitioner and family medicine in a multidisciplinary assessment clinic. While the relationships between nursing and family medicine were always positive, we built an increasingly trusting and shared collaborative interdependence, especially in relationship to the care of elderly patients. Moreover, the Committee on Aging implemented a Center on Healthy Aging. This Center, located in a shopping center in an area of town densely populated by the elderly, is a "one-stop shopping" approach to healthy aging. Nursing faculty significantly influenced the design, location, and most importantly, the philosophy of the Center on Healthy Aging, not an easy task. The Center recently received a Regional Educational Grant. In response to community needs, nurse practitioner faculty in the Center started an interdisciplinary Alzheimer Disease Support Group. Moreover, geriatric nurse practitioner faculty consulted with several acute care centers, and gained visiting privileges at several nursing homes which allowed them to follow patients and be reimbursed for visits to Center clients when they are admitted into a long-term care facility.

Thus, the TNHP extended the faculty's belief in practice and strengthened collegial relationships with clinicians from other disciplines. It improved their desire and ability to make a difference in the care of elderly nursing home patients, thereby improving their students' attitudes toward nursing home careers and encouraged them to involve themselves in legislative, political, and reimbursement issues. Perhaps most importantly, the TNHP enriched faculty research and scholarship regarding issues concerning the frail elderly. The TNHP strengthened the faculty's commitment to continuity of care, rehabilitation, and prevention and health promotion, especially with the elderly. The TNHP strengthened the faculty's enthusiasm and ability to make a difference in the functioning, morale, and discharge of elderly nursing home patients thereby improving students' attitudes toward nursing home practice. The TNHP strengthened the faculty's ability to involve themselves in legislative, political, and reimbursement issues. The TNHP strengthened the faculty's belief about research and clinical scholarship regarding issues concerning the frail elderly.

Most importantly, the faculty is convinced that community-linked systems of care developed for the elderly can serve as the prototype for emerging paradigms of health care delivery systems for the elderly, and for populations other than the elderly in need of continuous care.

TABLE 6.1 Health Care Delivery Paradigm Shift

Medical/Cure Model	Chronicity–Continuity Model
Disease based (deficits)	Need based (attributes)
High technology	Low technology
High specialization	Low specialization (paraprofessionals &
rigid Boundaries	volunteers)
fragmentation: Duplication	soft boundaries
	integrated
	multidisciplinary consultation
Episodic reimburse (KBF) revenue	Case-based reimburse (KBE)
	cost savings models
Patient centered	Family and social support centered
Hierarchy of decision	Interactional: collaborative/decisions
Appeals to authority	Empowers consumer/family decisions
Power of protected information	Power of shared information
Short-term planning:	Long-range planning: outcome oriented
Crisis management process oriented	

Recently, since assuming the position of Dean of the School of Nursing at the University of Rochester, I have had the opportunity to become immersed in a large acute, tertiary care center, and I have had time to reflect on the differences between systems which serve patients with acute conditions and systems whose primary purpose is chronic care. There is much to be learned about these differences.

The medical cure or "fix-it" model of acute care is disease and deficit based, while a chronicity–continuity model is need or attribute based (see Table 6.1). The primary intervention in acute care is high technology, while minimizing intrusive interventions to the client (low technology) is the goal in a continuity model.

The acute care model is highly bureaucratic, specialized, with turf issues, territoriality and rigid boundaries resulting in duplicating and fragmenting services. Continuity of care models require low specialization and bureaucracy, i.e., more advanced generalists, volunteers, family members and other support groups as care providers. While acute care is patient centered, continuity care is family and social support centered. It must have soft boundaries and an integrated matrix system of decentralized administration.

In the culture of acute care centers there exists a hierarchy of decision making, which appeals to bureaucratic authority. However, in a continuity-based model, interactive and collaborative decision making that involves consumers in the decision-making process is essential. There is abuse of power and refusal to share information in an acute or bureaucratic culture; power rests in shared information in the continuity model.

Finally, the reimbursement in cure models is individual and episodic; it operates from a principal called "keep the beds full." Though systems are rapidly moving toward case-based reimbursement, people have not yet reached an attitude of "let's keep the beds empty." As I see it, a fundamental dilemma facing nursing is how to demonstrate that quality nursing care yields cost savings rather than merely yielding new dollars or aiding budget neutrality. Nursing care does save dollars when and if the analysis includes all settings. However, at present, measurement of the cost of nursing care is usually confined to one setting at a time, thus we are rarely able to demonstrate how quality nursing care saves money throughout the system. Clients move through the health care system using resources; we need to show how nursing care facilitates a more efficient and effective use of resources. To do that, we need to fully understand the characteristics and implications of these two models, the acute care model *and* the continuity model; and, we need to demonstrate the essential components of nursing practice within these models.

Our experience convinces me that the TNHP served to empower nursing both internally and externally, it encouraged us to recommit our efforts to practice, research, and theory development. Nursing can and must take the lead in shaping the health care system for the elderly. A nursing orientation to care can provide the prototype for improving care not only for the elderly, but for other populations, for example, those with AIDS or with addictive, abusive, and violence disorders. Such patients may at times need the acute care setting for diagnosis and treatment but most of their care needs can be delivered within the community in the context of a continuity model. The TNHP gave nursing an opportunity to demonstrate its resolve and leadership in care of the elderly and gave all of us the opportunity to reflect on needed modifications across our health care system.

REFERENCES

1. Braden B et al. A conceptual scheme for the study of the etiology of pressure sores. *Rehabilitation Nursing* 1987; 12(1):8–12.
2. Herman J, & Krall K. University-sponsored home health care agency as a clinical site. *Image: J. Nurs Scholar* 1983; 16(3):77–75.
3. Foyt J. The functional status of elderly clients in eleven midwestern urban health maintenance clinics. Co-presented at the Nursing Research Forum sponsored by Creighton University School of Nursing Honor Society, Omaha, Neb., January 11, 1985.
4. Parsons C. Faculty practice in a nurse-managed center. Paper presented at the American Academy of Nursing, Clearwater Beach, FL, Third Faculty Practice Symposium, January 23, 1986.

CASE D
The Benjamin Rose Institute and the Frances Payne Bolton School of Nursing, Case Western Reserve University: The Nursing Home Administrator's Perspective

Alice J. Kethley

The Robert Wood Johnson Teaching Nursing Home Program provided academic institutions and skilled nursing facilities with an incentive to join together for the purpose of addressing some of the issues associated with the delivery of long-term care, one of the most problematic areas in health care today.

The Need for Well-Prepared Nurses in the Nursing Home Setting: When Medicare introduced its hospital reimbursement policy in 1983, the role of nurses working in nursing homes began to change dramatically. Medicare policy sought to reduce hospital costs and succeeded in cutting the number of hospital days by building in an incentive for earlier discharge. This was accomplished by discharging patients earlier to nursing homes (or home health agencies). The staff in nursing homes were not prepared to provide the care needed by this new client group.

Historically, the nursing home industry had provided for the elderly who needed low-tech care and personal care. Nurses who did not enjoy the high-tech environment of hospitals had turned to nursing homes as a career alternative because of the emphasis on "hands-on care."

Not so long ago, nursing homes were fighting the image of "warehousing" and were not recognized as part of the health care system. Curriculum in schools of nursing did not include care for nursing home residents. Nurses who worked in nursing homes were not considered to be "the best." The sudden change to discharging hospitalized elderly patients to nursing homes as part of their recovery from an acute medical episode or surgery made it necessary that nursing home staff nurses be retrained in procedures which generally had not been used in nursing homes. The Teaching Nursing Home Program was well timed in that it offered the opportunity for nurses to address the changing role of the nurse in a skilled nursing facility.

The successes and the problems encountered by one of the participating skilled facilities—the Margaret Wagner Home of the Benjamin Rose

Institute—are discussed in this chapter. The Robert Wood Johnson Teaching Nursing Home Program was a joint venture between two of Cleveland's most respected organizations: The Frances Payne Bolton School of Nursing of Case Western Reserve University and The Benjamin Rose Institute. Benjamin Rose and Case Western have a long history of working together collaborating to address the educational, clinical, and research issues in the fields of geriatrics and gerontology. In 1953, The Benjamin Rose Institute built a small geriatric teaching and research hospital on the Case Western campus to encourage nursing, medical, and other professionals into the field. The Institute viewed the Teaching Nursing Home Program as an excellent opportunity to join the School of Nursing in addressing common concerns regarding the quality of long-term care in a residential setting. To improve the quality of care, the School and the Institute established several activities:

1. Rotation of bachelor and master's level students through Margaret Wagner House for clinical training in a nursing home committed to high quality care;
2. Testing new and innovative clinical procedures developed by participating faculty, Margaret Wagner House staff, and students;
3. Research conducted by faculty, students, and Margaret Wagner House staff in order to improve efficiency and quality of care;
4. Examination and development of new procedures to improve operation of the Home, and;
5. Development and testing of educational materials appropriate for in-service training which could be replicated in long-term care facilities.

Margaret Wagner House and the School of Nursing were within walking distance of each other. This convenient location facilitated staff, faculty, and students' collaboration in these activities.

Benjamin Rose Institute: Its Advantages to the Program

The most important advantage that the Benjamin Rose Institute offered the Teaching Nursing Home Program was Margaret Wagner House, a 175-bed skilled nursing facility. The occupancy rate is approximately 94%. All beds are certified as skilled, but residents' needs range from total care to assisted living (4%). Among the Home's many special programs are a Protective Care Unit for cognitively impaired, a short-term rehabilitation program an adult day care program, and a respite care program.

The Institute's research division, the Margaret Blenkner Research Center, provides the nursing home staff with consultation and support. For example, the research staff worked with the nursing staff to develop a computer program to analyze residents' care plans. They also assisted in revising forms, designing research projects, and writing proposals. The Research Center staff worked with clinical staff to develop measures for evaluating new programs and procedures.

The Community Services Division of the Institute provided another advantage to the Project. The director of the Institute's certified home health care program, who is an adjunct faculty member of the School of Nursing, taught students about the interface between nursing home care and home health care. The relationship between these two types of care became increasingly important since the Home's short-term rehabilitative program had increased short-term stays in the facility, and discharge planning was necessary. The use of a skilled nursing facility in this way is appropriate but necessitates that nurses have a better understanding of home health care vis-à-vis nursing home care. Short-term residents from Margaret Wagner House may choose either in-home services from our home health care division, out-patient rehabilitation services, or adult day care at Margaret Wagner House. Whatever type of service is chosen by the residents and their families, nurses are needed who understand and can implement the system of care.

The Institute supported the Teaching Nursing Home Project not only with its divisions, but also with funds. We recognized that the goals of the Foundation were compatible with the mission of the Institute, and therefore, supported three half-time positions (.5 F.T.E.) and one 40% (.4 F.T.E.) position. The director of nursing was the only previously existing position and that position was upgraded to a masters-prepared nurse for purposes of the project. After the program ended, these positions have continued by joint agreement with the School of Nursing.

One other advantage that the Benjamin Rose Institute brought to the Teaching Nursing Home Program was its interest and commitment. In carrying out our mission to provide the highest quality of services and to promote the independence and dignity of our residents, we are equally concerned with our employees. The Teaching Nursing Home Program gave us the opportunity to address some of the negative factors that affect nurses and others who work in the nursing home setting. Our goal was not only to attract nurses to work at Margaret Wagner House, but also to improve the work environment through more efficient strategies of care that would provide more worker satisfaction as well as better patient care. Employee satisfaction means a higher quality of care for our residents.

Curriculum for Nurses: A Nursing Home Perspective

The Teaching Nursing Home Program made clear a number of educational needs in long-term nursing. The following suggestions for the nursing curriculum are presented from the nursing home perpective and may differ slightly from the academic view. First, a discreet curriculum of nursing home care and administration must be included in the nursing program. If nurses are to consider long-term care facilities as a viable career alternative, coursework and clinical training must be available. Geriatrics and gerontology programs seem a logical place for such education. The strategy of "getting to students while they are young" proved successful with other professional fields which had difficulty attracting students. The demographic trends of a rapidly growing elderly population and a dwindling supply of future nurses make the need for such training essential.

The Teaching Nursing Home experience at Margaret Wagner House also gave us some definite ideas concerning additions to the curriculum, over and above the already superb preparation in clinical practice procedures. Nurses in the nursing home setting serve in supervisory positions. They work in conjunction with nursing assistants who provide the "hands on" personal care (bathing, feeding, dressing, walking, etc.). The use of these paraprofessionals helps to contain the cost of nursing home care. The nurse must oversee these aides and orchestrate their varied activities. Nursing home residents are generally sick and incapable of doing for themselves so the nurse must supervise an environment of constant caregiving—bed changing, assisting with toileting, helping up, helping down, dressing, undressing, etc. Nurses in these supervisory roles require training that prepares them to motivate staff, manage conflict among staff as well as between staff and residents, supervise staff with different racial and cultural backgrounds, and deal with staff stress. The skill with which a nurse is able to perform these and other supervisory functions sets the tone of the nursing home.

Unlike hospitals, the nursing home setting does not have many technical and staff supports. Physicians are highly visible and primary decisionmakers in hospitals but not in nursing homes. Nurses find that in nursing homes not only is there little or no physician input, but fewer and often no other nurses are present to share in decision making. The nurse, thus, finds that she makes more decisions about interventions or procedures to deal with resident problems. The lack of on-site professional consultation indicates the need for additional preparation. Nurses must know how to communicate clearly, concisely, and assertively with physicians concerning residents. This is particularly important when there is limited direct nurse/physician contact. Importantly, this should include coursework that prepares the nurse for clinical decisionmaking in a setting without on-site medical and technical backup.

Hospitals are large institutions with a regular turnover of patients, a mobile staff, and places to "hide." Nursing homes have limited space, long-term residents, and few places where staff members can get away. The nursing home environment demands good communication skills and even better interpersonal skills. A nursing home can be challenging to well-prepared nurses who quickly learn the important role they play in such an environment. The nurse can promote an atmosphere of dignity and choice for residents in an institutional setting.

The director of nursing should thoroughly understand the business aspects of nursing homes. Most nurses who move from the acute care setting to the long-term care setting are surprised at the extent to which the reimbursement systems of Medicare and medicaid control and regulate the care. In Ohio, visits from the standard/certifying branch can be quite disruptive if the documentation and procedures are not prepared in advance. While knowledge of reimbursement systems is desirable, knowledge of how to prepare staff for government scrutiny is more important. The nursing home industry is highly regulated, because it is also part of the business of long-term care. Reimbursement requires meticulous recordkeeping. In this electronic age, nursing care plans are best recorded on computers. We have to teach nursing students to become computer friendly early in their professional education.

Attitudes and concepts about the elderly must be introduced into the nursing curriculum. The needs of nursing home residents extend much farther than their obvious need for personal care and health monitoring. Through academic programs, students could be made aware of the mental health needs of both the residents and their families. Many families are actively involved in caring for an elderly family member in the home. Nurses should understand the family caregiver needs and the role a family which is very helpful or very disruptive can play. The family will turn to the nurse for assurance and guidance.

Working together, we should offer a broad view of nursing home care which will encourage students to consider nursing homes as a career path that offers opportunity for clinical practice and research. In the process, we will create a more positive attitude toward nursing homes as a legitimate and integral part of the health care system.

Problems Encountered During the Teaching Nursing Home Program

Frequently faculty and staff viewed the problems associated with the program as challenges. At the outset it was feared that student rotation might disturb the residents and disrupt the nursing home routine. Staff soon recognized that the Home's routine was enhanced as students successfully tested new ideas.

A more difficult problem, associated with a limited number of individual faculty and staff, was coordinating the roles between the two institutions. The program worked best when faculty viewed themselves as clinical specialists associated with Margaret Wagner House. Those faculty play a valuable clinical and consultant role to the Home. The problem was with a limited number of faculty who were not willing to spend time at the Home. These faculty seemed to regard the nursing home as merely a convenient setting for their research and case studies. However, most faculty and staff associated with the program became very involved with the challenges presented by both the teaching of students and the quest for ways of improving care in the Home.

Some day-to-day problems surfaced because of the age of the facility. Because Margaret Wagner House first opened in 1961, adequate parking for today's auto-rich workforce, student groups, and faculty does not exist. The Home also lacks sufficient office space for students or faculty to work and to hold conferences. This shortage of space proved irritating and served as an excuse for not spending more time on site. Seminars, group meetings, and larger classes had to be scheduled carefully around the Home's normal activities. The facility was stretched to its utmost capacity to accommodate the extra people involved in the program, the actual crowding provided the reality of the nursing home setting. Working in the nursing home environment does not allow for a great deal of privacy. Modern Nursing homes are constructed to maximize staff's ability to see (and be seen) so that they can monitor residents.

The Benjamin Rose Institute is a charitable organization which considers the education of professionals "in the art of serving the elderly" to be part of its mission. We were not surprised that being part of the Teaching Nursing Home Program added to our cost of care. Just as teaching hospitals incur extra expense for the clinical education of medical and other students, so do nursing homes, and the expense comes in a variety of forms. It is staff time working with students, or time spent addressing problems that occur when clinical practice is combined with research and teaching. Sometimes it is the cost of hiring staff at the masters level in order to meet academic requirements for the supervision of graduate and undergraduate students. The issue should not be the expense of nursing education, but rather how to pay for a valid and needed program. It is evident that at this time nursing homes cannot add educational expense to the cost of service as teaching hospitals do.

The partnership between the academic community and a community nursing home requires commitment from the upper administrative levels of both institutions. Formal lines of communication must be established and used throughout the program. As their first task, participating staff and faculty should develop a procedure manual that covers such topics as utilization of residents for research purposes, utilization of space, involvement of staff in teaching, and other vital activities. New items should be added to the manual as issues arise and are resolved. It is very difficult to maintain an atmosphere of equality if those who are affected most by the activities of the Project's nursing home staff do not understand what the rules and procedures are. A second-class citizenship phenomenon occurs when those who work at the facility every day find their schedules rearranged to accommodate the needs of those who seem to come and go at will—students and faculty. Nursing home staff members do not get semester or quarter breaks, four days vacation for Thanksgiving, or spring vacation. A procedure manual that covers sensitive areas such as these would diffuse the feelings among nursing home staff that the program exploited the resources of the nursing home without equal return.

Positive Outcomes of the Program

Positive outcomes of the Teaching Nursing Home Program far outnumbered the drawbacks. The best evidence of its success is that The Benjamin Rose Institite is willing to continue its support after the program ended. Margaret Wagner House benefited greatly in terms of education opportunities for its staff. Margaret Wagner nurses were given many opportunities to earn CEUs in classes organized around educational needs of staff which had been identified by the Program. Students doing their rotation at Margaret Wagner House were very helpful in providing special training to nursing assistants. Evening seminars were offered at the Home, and staff from other parts of the Institute were invited as well as people from the community. The evening seminars provided an opportunity for researchers and educators not actively involved in the project to present their work.

Many of the research projects resulted in new programs; for example, a study on falls among the residents was published. More important to resident care, the study led to the development of a mobility program for residents prone to fallling. A training program showed staff how to identify potential fallers and how to work with them. Walking schedules were developed for residents considered prone to falling to insure that they had the exercise so vital to overall well-being.

One faculty member who became extremely interested in our Protective Care Unit conducted a number of studies. Her study on the effect of noise on demented and confused individuals found that loud and unusual noise led to agitated and disruptive behavior. We are therefore taking measures to reduce noise in the protective care unit. Likewise, studies of temperature, staffing patterns, and staff stress led to adaptations and plans which will ameliorate working and living conditions in the unit. A student project resulted in an ongoing current events program in which a nursing assistant reviews the Cleveland Plain Dealer with residents daily.

Infection control is an ongoing problem in many institutional settings. One contribution of the program was the monitoring of areas most likely to harbor infection-causing bacteria (century whirlpool tubs, physical therapy whirlpool, resident floors, etc.). Educational programs on hand washing and other procedures helped to raise staff consciousness about the problem by revising and distributing a hygiene guide to the staff as a reminder and reference. Incidents of infection declined and, more importantly, the entire staff became more aware of simple procedures which would help reduce infection.

As a result of the Teaching Nursing Home program, a clinical specialist was added to the staff. The position was funded equally by the School of Nursing and Margaret Wagner House. The clinical specialist serves as a consultant to nurses and to rehabilitation staff in the House, as well as a liaison between the House and hospitals. The clinical specialist worked with hospital discharge planners and families to determine whether Margaret Wagner House was an appropriate placement for the elderly patient. The clinical specialist developed the procedures for admitting short-term rehabilitation residents into the Home and coordinated the interdisciplinary short-term rehabilitation team. The benefits of having a clinical specialist (a masters-prepared clinician with special training in geriatric care) are very evident. The real issue is whether or not nursing homes can afford such a position. We are continuing the clinical specialist position, but we are concerned about the budgetary implications in a underfinanced health care setting.

The baccalaureate and master level students who completed their clinical rotations at Margaret Wagner House became a source of part-time and even a few full-time staff nurses. They and we had positive student experiences. We were able to match our labor needs with student financial needs to develop schedules to mutually benefit students and the nursing home. We found it very helpful to have a pool of nurses, familiar with the residents and routine of the Home, and willing to work.

Is There a Future?

The Teaching Nursing Home Program ended in May 1987. Despite the willingness of the Benjamin Rose Institute to maintain its financial support, it has been difficult to keep the program going. An agency such as ours has an ongoing commitment to find solutions to the issues which surround long-term older adult care services.

Our mission is to continue to implement better and more efficient clinical practice strategies; to foster and conduct research on all aspects of nursing home and community service; and to provide education for our own staff through in-service collaborative training efforts with educational institutions. The Institute is single minded in its efforts; academic institutions are not. Faculty are free, and rightly so, to pursue research and teaching activities and to create new knowledge of their own interest. An agency must respond to the needs of the clients and its community. A university creates its own community. It is difficult to maintain a program such as the Teaching Nursing Home Program once the financial incentive for the academician ends.

The Program succeeded in converting some faculty to research and teaching related to long-term care, although others have already returned to their original areas of interst. Margaret Wagner House, like many other nursing homes across the country, is advertising for staff nurses but with little success. The Program did succeed in increasing the number of baccalaureate and masters prepared nurses in nursing home care. The research articles published as a result of the Program have benefited the field and yes, Margaret Wagner House would do it again.

Long-term care, whether in an institution or in the home, will continue to be a major problem for the health care industry. It is still questionable whether or not nurses in an academic setting will become leaders in finding solutions to the problems of long-term quality care. It is a frontier beset with historical problems. The Robert Wood Johnson Foundation Teaching Nursing Home Program was a tentative first step nursing homes and schools of nursing must take to find solutions to long-term care problem.

7

The Nursing Profession and Reform of Service for the Elderly

Rosemary Stevens

American nursing in the late nineteenth and early twentieth centuries was a young profession bent on reform. Nurses championed the reform of hospitals, maternal and child health, and pioneered so many of the health and social reforms that today are taken for granted. Today, that proud heritage—nurse as reformer—has particular relevance for the profession. There must be someone to speak for the institutionalized old-old and the frail elderly who are part of the nation's fastest growing population, those aged 65 and over. No group is more in need of champions. No group is more able to champion their cause then nursing. And there is no better pulpit than nursing homes.

As a historian, I wish to focus on two basic points: (1) that the nursing home concept which first originated in the 1960s is highly susceptible to change through federal policy and regulation, state policy, and media pressure; and (2) that nursing homes present an ideal target for reform by nurses through organizational pressure. I do not mean to imply that nurses are either the obvious or only group concerned with nursing home reform. On the contrary, consumer advocates, social workers, and other major lobbying groups have been far more vocal in expressing a strong opinion on nursing home issues than have nurses. This is even more surprising, considering that there are 1.8 million nurses, the single largest professional group within the health care industry. The enormous potential clout of such a large group, coupled with the growing national visibility of the elderly as voters and lobbyists, has tremendous implications for reform.

Nursing Home History: Federal Policy/Tangled Threads

The history of nursing homes in American society is essentially one of change. The modern nursing home concept had its earliest beginnings in the 1930s when widows' pensions, the Social Security Act of 1935, and Old Age Assistance first became available to the elderly. With those new resources, the aged found that they no longer had to depend solely on the county farms and poor houses which were often degrading warehouses for the sick. Private homes for those who had at least limited resources began to spring up. Then, even as now, American nursing home policy was distinguished by money, that is, by the purchasing power of the consumer, rather than by strategies for optimal care.

Funds for nursing home care have invariably been associated with relatively indigent individuals. Although the Social Security Act enlarged the pool of those who could afford some type of boarding care, these people generally were at the lower end of the socioeconomic scale. Federal vendor medical payments, approved in 1950, were based on similar assumptions.

Nursing homes thus have had three basic antecedents: public almshouses, voluntary homes for the aged, and private boarding homes for indigent adults. The United States has never had a standardized nursing home system, that is, a system designed to care for all members of the population on an equal basis. Nor was there, prior to Medicare and Medicaid, any standard definition for what a nursing home was. Many nursing home owners and administrators backed into the field. For instance, those who had taken one or several elderly persons into their home for personal care found, that over time, some of their guests became ill and there was nowhere to send them. Thus homeowners became nursing home owners by default.

In the late 1960s, when Medicare and Medicaid were implemented, there was a hodgepodge of institutions under the nursing home umbrella, with no clear definition of either role or purpose. To compound the problem, nursing homes had negative connotations in the American context associated with both age and indigence.

Nursing homes in New Hampshire in the 1960s provide an example of the overall situation in general. A 1965 state survey showed that there were 169 nursing homes with close to 5,000 beds. The typical patient was an eighty-year-old widow. One of every four residents was on welfare. The facilities ranged from skilled nursing homes to residential homes for the aged. Collectively, the homes were akin to a cottage industry, similar to the early forms of day care for children. Approximately 50% of the homes were operated by people with an RN or LPN diploma. The remainder were operated by people with a wide variety of backgrounds: housewives, nursing home aides, store owners, as well as former teachers, construction workers, salesmen, and so on. Most of these homes were "proprietary" in the old sense, that is, they had been started by a proprietor.

This situation began to change and change rapidly after Medicare and Medicaid came into being. Because their reimbursement policies were limited to medical rather than social care, nursing homes were required to distinguish between their nursing and nonnursing functions. In retrospect, there is a certain irony in the rapidity with which rules and regulations for certification were developed. With both Medicare and Medicaid hard at work dividing medical from nonmedical functions, at least for the indigent, there was a rapid acceptance of different nursing home functions (Skilled Nursing Facility, Intermediate Nursing Facility, neither) that was based on the level of *sickness* of the patient. It seems somewhat incongruous that today life-care homes and similar arrangements are reinventing the combination, that is, combining residential and nursing care for affluent Americans. For most Americans, however, federal policy has narrowed the definition of nursing home care.

The nursing home problem in the 1960s was not only one of definition but also of money. Federal policy indirectly was pushing nursing homes into corporate arrangements. Hill-Burton funds, for example, were limited to voluntary or governmental organizations, even though most nursing homes were proprietary. Proprietary homes, in turn, sought loans from the Small Business Administration or from the private sector. These economic expediencies caused proprietors to see themselves as business operators and accelerated the move to incorporate. The stage was set for the rapid expansion of the profit-making sector in the nursing home field, as the health care industry began to respond to the realities of Medicare and Medicaid.

Medicare and Medicaid: Protection for Income, Not Health Care

Medicare and Medicaid posed new problems for the nursing home field by requiring standard definitions for functions and facilities. Individual differences in purpose between the two programs compounded the problems.

Medicare was, in effect, an income protection program designed to protect the elderly from enormous hospital bills incurred in catastrophic illnesses. Nursing homes for extended care, that is, nonhospital facilities that provided skilled nursing and rehabilitation on a daily basis, provided neither convalescent care nor residential care.

What Medicare actually did was to emphasize the role of the nursing home as a *skilled* nursing facility, while ignoring the other functions and services traditionally associated with nursing home. It is significant that in the Medicare lexicon, "skill" was assumed to be quasi-hospital care.

Federal regulations for Medicaid also required states to provide skilled nursing facilities and, later, intermediate care facilities. The Medicaid program, so important in fueling both the demand and supply of nursing home beds, also promulgated the role of nursing homes as homes for the *indigent*. Through a perverse logic, Medicaid has effectively pauperized many elderly through its spend-down provisions for nursing home care. Since the typical nursing home resident today is an elderly widow, Medicaid has reinforced the prevailing public image of the nursing home as a warehouse for the (mostly white) elderly who are socially dependent.

Medicare and Medicaid had a combined impact that shifted the balance of income in nursing homes. In 1965, 65% of all nursing home income came from private funds, mostly all out-of-pocket. By the late 1970s, most of the reimbursement for nursing home care came from public sources.

Government became responsible for nursing home care through a process of policy drift. In effect, however, no government agency was directly in charge. The federal government could claim that the states had the responsibility for running the Medicaid programs. The state, in turn, could say that their role was only to purchase care in the private sector. The overriding purpose of both programs has been to protect the income of the elderly, to contain hospital (and more recently nursing home) costs, and to regulate reimbursement which stresses basic standards. But neither Medicare nor Medicaid has assumed any ethical responsibility for the quality of long-term care of the elderly.

Nursing homes at present comprise a large industry of small units. The United States has over 19,000 nursing homes with an average of 85 beds per home. Three-fourths of the homes are proprietary institutions. It is interesting to note that nursing homes are still described as "proprietary" while hospitals are "investor owned." The most recent phenomena in the nursing home industry are the new nursing home chains and the affiliations between nursing homes, hospitals, and HMOs. Of the 19,000 homes across the nation, 41% currently belong to nursing home chains.

Nursing home care is expensive. In 1985, private patients paid an average $61 a day for skilled care. Federal policy has driven up costs in the name of quality, yet nursing homes are constantly denigrated and criticized as places to be avoided if any other choice is available. Economically and socially, modern nursing homes are the end product of government incentives.

Who Is to Speak for—and about—the Elderly?

The 83,000 registered nurses who work in nursing homes appear at first glance an ideal group to lobby for nursing home reform. Yet this relatively large group of health professionals encompass only 10% of nursing home employees. The remaining 90%, LPNs, nursing aides, and orderlies, perform most of the personal care services for the residents of the home. Moreover, due to the small size of most of the homes, there are only a few registered nurses in each institution.

Consensus regarding the appropriate role of registered nurses in a nursing home in terms of management, supervision, clinical work, bedside nursing, and patient advocacy has not been reached. Because of problems of dispersion and role definition, nursing has been unable (or unwilling) to speak with one voice on behalf of the elderly.

The nursing viewpoint is also essential if we are to change society's assumptions about nursing homes and the elderly. The root cause of the major misperceptions of the nation's elderly nursing home population is ageism. Ageism—prejudice against the elderly—persists despite the efforts to suppress it and sometimes seemingly helpful information is presented in a way that sustains our deepest prejudices.

For example, in a recent report, the National Center for Health Statistics (NCHS) noted that urinary incontinence is "a common medical problem among older individuals." Yet the same NCHS report found that among the general population, 94% of those aged 65–74 years, and 87% of those aged 75 years and older, have *no* problem of incontinence. The percentages cause one to wonder why NCHS would term urinary incontinence "a common problem."

Another distressing misperception is the association of old age with sickness, despite the fact that most of the elderly population function well. The data shows that 62% of all those aged 75 years and over reported no days in bed in the past year. Over 50% of those aged 85 years and over reported no hearing impairment; nearly 75% reported no visual impairment. In short, the aged population generally functions well, yet the association of age with sickness persists.

Finally, nursing homes have a strongly negative public image in comparison with hospitals. Both, in some ways, are associated with "failure" for these are the places where people go when their health is impaired. Yet hospitals, because of the enormous value that society places on "science," are viewed optimistically as progressive institutions, whereas nursing homes continue to be associated with the image of the poor and dependent elderly.

Why should the nursing home not serve as a center for teaching, research, and service for the healthy older population in the same way that the hospital does for the population in general? The answer is that it should. This brings me to the most important point—the relationship between the nursing profession and nursing home in the years to come.

The Future: Nursing Homes as a Vehicle for Professional Development

Doctors and nurses learn from the sick, and are supposed to apply what they have learned to serving the healthy as well. The principle, incongruous as it may seem, is well-accepted. Teaching nursing homes follow the same general principle: what is learned from the care of the frail elderly will ultimately have implications for the well elderly. But the teaching nursing home concept offers a new twist, as I will explain.

In the past, doctors and nurses have not shaped hospital service in terms of wider health care needs. Instead, hospitals have been shaped by the dual drives of capital and reimbursement, as expressed in the managerial policies of hospital executives, physicians, and trustees. The teaching nursing home is the ideal setting for nurses to assume professional leadership in teaching and research—leadership that is unfettered by narrowly defined teaching and research expectations that hospitals have shaped over the years.

The teaching nursing home has enormous potential as a model of what a nursing home should be, given the constraints of resources, how the nursing home should fit with other elements in the health care system. Teaching nursing homes can be used to explore and articulate institutional philosophies. They can be working laboratories for patient care where nursing knowledge is applied; a place where questions can be posed, such as to what degree the intellectual (and sexual) capacities of all residents should be maintained in order to provide the best individual life experiences. They should provide a basis for nursing gerontological research that includes not only research based within the home, but also community-based studies, including links with social services and rehabilitation.

More widely, the teaching nursing home should provide an important conceptual break with the medical mystique: redefining aspects of health care, including nursing, as reform. Reform, in this sense, has two meanings: (1) reform in Medicare and Medicaid that would address the problems of the elderly more directly, and (2) push for nursing in the 1990s to be identified with improved quality of life for the aged.

The teaching nursing home program is still in its infancy and all of its many possibilities have yet to be explored. It would be sad if the program were to be a model that merely tinkered with the status quo and accepted Medicare and Medicaid as given. I raise this caveat because merely reviewing the role of teaching nursing homes in academic centers or merely reviewing teaching, research, and nursing practice within existing nursing home parameters seems dangerously tame. Why should patients' needs and society's priorities be an irreconcilable dilemma? That brings us back to the question of who sets the priorities for society and the more fundamental issues of power, influence, and money.

Someone suggested to me that nurses see themselves as a marginal profession and nursing home patients as marginal members of society. I found both statements shocking. Nurses have potentially great power which they have yet to exercise fully. They can demonstrate this power through professional organizations and nursing schools, through networks of nurse executives in health care chains and major hospitals, through congressional committees and foundations, and through individual leverage within existing organizations. Are nurses now pressing, for example, for redirection of the money flow within major corporate budgets? Within state Medicaid programs? Or in Medicare? Some are. More could. Why are nurses politically timid?

Nursing home patients must not be regarded as marginal. A huge sector of the American population is vitally concerned about the issue of nursing home care, whether for themselves, their parents and relatives, or their friends. Mid-life crisis stems from an apprehension about the future and the likelihood of being a candidate for nursing home care. In short, there is a very large interest group, strongly represented in the American Association for Retired People (AARP) for whom nursing homes are an important item on the middle class agenda. Nursing homes are *not* an issue that only concerns the indigent. Nor do people want to become indigent because they require nursing home care.

Finally, and most importantly, teaching nursing homes offer the nursing profession a strategic battleground from which they can lead the fight for better medical care and health for everyone.

The final outcome rests with nursing. Will nurses sit back and let others make decisions? Or will nurses remember the profession's management and political roles in its early days and become, once again, effective advocates for health? There can be no better pulpit than the teaching nursing home.

8

Involving Nurse Educators in Gerontology and Geriatrics

Jean R. Miller

Health has the greatest impact on the quality of life for older individuals, yet we as a society have been slow to respond to the needs of our frail elderly. My purpose is to describe (1) the responsibilities of health professionals *in academe* in meeting the needs of the dependent elderly, (2) the means by which health professionals can be prepared to meet these needs, (3) marketing strategies that will increase social awareness of resources available for the frail elderly, and (4) the rewards for service in gerontology.

Responsibilities of Health Professionals

The mission of a university is to meet the needs of society through teaching, research, and service . . . and society includes the old as well as the young. Part of our mission then is to improve the quality of life of the elderly, and we can do this only if we can effect change in society and its institutions. Education is our most powerful tool for it is the aim of education according to McMurrin, to "conserve, criticize, improve, and perpetuate social institutions" (and) contribute to the achievement of authentic individuality and the well-being of the individual." These goals are particularly relevant to the needs of the elderly in our society.

Faculty in university health schools are strategically positioned to respond to the needs of the frail elderly. Through our teaching and research, we can change society's attitudes about priorities of care for the elderly. Through our knowledge, skills, and values, we can prepare students for professional practice that will improve the quality of life for aged patients.

Multidisciplinary Nursing Home Teams

Multidisciplinary teams are ideally suited to care of the frail elderly for these patients have complex medical, behavioral, and social problems.[1] The basic nursing home team consists of the patient, a baccalaureate nurse, a physician, a pharmacist, and a social worker. The characteristics of the nursing home team resemble those of any other team, that is, a group of individuals who (1) have common goals and are accountable to one another, (2) assume a division of responsibility and power, and (3) has an integral communications system.[2] In the health care model, meeting the needs of the patient is the common goal, and the team members, including the patient, participate according to their individual ability and skill. Although the patient holds the ultimate power, the whole team, rather than any individual member, shares in decision making.

A successful team can be easily identified. The members share a sense of belonging and the awareness that their ideas are being heard, accepted, and respected. They exchange their opinions, insights, and feelings, and they accept their differences. They hold their achievements in common, even though some may have contributed more than others.[3] Most of all, they are effective. Research has shown that the greater the collegiality, the more positive the outcomes for the team, patient and professionals alike.[4]

Nurses' Role in Nursing Home Teams

Many nursing home teams choose to have the professional nurse assume the major role in coordinating the care of patients, because the nurse generally spends the most time with the elderly residents. The nurse-coordinator must be skilled in group processes and communication, and must know what services are being provided by the other team members and what resources and patient support systems are available. The nurse must also be able to determine when it is necessary to call the team together.[5]

The nurse on the team also provides direct care for the elderly patients. In its best expression, this is the goal of nursing: "caring which protects, enhances, and preserves human dignity."[6] Caring allows the patient to generate inner strength that facilitates healing of the mind, body, and spirit. The caring nurse possesses good listening skills to "hear" what the patient says and means, and possesses sound clinical judgment and related skills integrated into nursing's heritage of wholism, the metaphysical aspects of the person-nurse interaction, and the artistic dimensions of nursing.

Faculty Development in the Care of the Frail Elderly

We cannot have effective nursing home teams unless we as faculty members first have the appropriate knowledge, skills, and attitudes regarding care for the frail elderly. Unfortunately, most nurses, academicians, and practitioners alike have only limited clinical experience in long-term care institutions. Too often, our clinical experience in nursing homes has been one of making beds and giving baths rather than learning the skills needed to care for the highly specific needs of elderly patients.

Fortunately, there are a few who recognize the critical need for health professionals prepared to care for the infirm elderly. The Robert Wood Johnson Foundation includes some of these forward thinkers. Among the objectives of this Teaching Nursing Home Program was maturation of knowledge, skills, and attitudes of the professionals and nursing home administrators who participated. This is also one of the goals of the research-focused teaching nursing home projects funded by the National Institute on Aging. Postdoctoral fellowships in gerontological nursing are yet another means of increasing faculty knowledge about the elderly patient.

As nursing school faculty, we must also take the lead in generating knowledge and teaching skills related to the care of the elderly. Some effective strategies that we might use include seminars and workshops led by experts in the field, faculty representation at gerontological meetings, the use of audiovisual resources, and expanded collections of gerontological journals and books in our university libraries. These activities could be opportunities for nursing and other health science faculty members to learn to work together with elderly patients. Students could have no better role models for multidisciplinary relationships than health professionals who work together.

Curriculum: Nursing Care for the Elderly

The curriculum of all health disciplines must keep pace with the new knowledge in gerontology. The criteria for gerontological content in the curriculum are determined by the clinical practices expected of the graduates as well as the information, skills, and attitudes needed to attain this goal. Decisions concerning the integration of gerontology into the curriculum must be made politically and rationally. The decision process itself may be different in each institution, but all institutions should have as broad a spectrum of faculty participation as possible. Broad participation in decisionmaking also helps faculty members to understand why certain gerontological content is important and essential. Furthermore, decisions about the curriculum give faculty a personal stake in the results, enhance collegiality, and increase faculty self-worth.[7]

In university schools of nursing, we often use the lecture to teach gerontological content, regardless of the level of knowledge being presented, the types of skills being taught, or the attitudes being conveyed. I would suggest that ideally a variety of methods should be used. For example, if we want students to synthesize knowledge in the care of the elderly, we should present the knowledge through examples that require synthesis rather than through rote information. Our examinations should test the ability of students to gather a variety of information, assemble it, and reach accurate conclusions. We should help our students learn skills through hands-on experience, not just in the laboratory but primarily in practice with patients. Attitudinal instruction is crucial in a society full of stereotypes about the aged. Students will learn respect for the elderly most effectively from a professor who demonstrates respect in his or her own relationships with the aged and in discussions of gerontological problems.

Gerontological Nursing Research

Gerontological nursing research is the basis for curriculum content and practice. It is the foundation for actions that can make the difference in the quality of life for the elderly. Whether society decides to make health care of the frail elderly a high priority will depend in large part on the quality and quantity of nursing research in the area.

As nurse researchers, we must study issues that are important to the wellbeing of patients, and we must use methodology appropriate for those issues. For example, many issues that concern patient well-being are at the initial level of inquiry, and questions such as "What is this?" are appropriate. At the next level of inquiry, we should be concerned with "What's happening here?" These two questions generally describe a situation and therefore lend themselves to exploratory or descriptive research design. Once we ask the initial questions, we can move forward to correlational, survey, experimental, and predictive designs.

Here the questions concern "What will happen if . . .?" or "How can I make . . . happen?"[8]

At the initial level of exploration, the most appropriate research methods are qualitative: We elicit information from the patient and the family by providing limited predetermined cues. In this way, we gain the true meaning of an issue from the perspective of the patient, rather than from the perspective of the researcher. Qualitative methods are gaining acceptance but nurse researchers accustomed to experimental designs and quantitative measures may find them difficult to use.

Measurement of behavior, feelings, and attitudes requires further development. Presently, nurse researchers have to use instruments already tested on other populations, and these may not be as reliable for elderly populations. Research designs and methods of analysis must incorporate multiple variables since heterogeneous variables affect the quality of life of the elderly. Experimental designs that ignore complicating factors do not present an accurate picture of the variables that affect the physiology, behavior, and attitudes of the aged. Multiple variables must be considered even in relatively clear-cut experimental designs if we are to present an accurate picture of the main effects. Multivariate analyses also may incorporate aspects of complex mind-body relationships which currently are being investigated. Returning to an earlier theme, the need to examine multiple variables that affect quality of life for the elderly underscores the importance of a multidisciplinary approach.

Marketing Strategies

Our university schools of nursing can and do produce graduates who deliver services to the frail elderly. But a cadre of prepared health professionals is only a first step in meeting their many needs. Positions with competitive pay must be available so that these professionals can practice. Such a market presupposes a demand and there can be a demand for these health care services only if the public is aware of their availablity. It is vital to educate long-term care administrators to demand well-prepared nurses to fill positions in nursing homes. Families and nursing home residents need to learn that they can expect more from nursing.

Marketing Analysis

Marketing health care begins by knowing what the consumers need. Health professionals must satisfy those needs and provide services that benefit patients and their families. However, fiscal restraints make it essential that we identify target health care consumer groups, those in greatest need of care. We may then define each of these groups by the number of persons with a specific problem, the group's rate of growth, and the profitability in serving this particular group. Profitability, in this context, means not only remuneration but also the physical and emotional outcomes which result from the services of health professionals.[9]

Ethics enter into the decision of whom should be given services. Some believe that all frail elderly have a right to care, but the economy and values of society do not permit *all* elderly to have equal access to care. Presently, those who can afford to pay are those who receive services. As the positive outcomes of gerontological care become evident, society may begin to reassess it's priorities and national budget so that all can receive care.

Communication Strategies

We need a communication strategy to market the services of the gerontological nursing team so that society will want to purchase health care services for the frail elderly. We first must make society aware that such services are available, and then explain the benefit of clinical interventions with the frail elderly. This new awareness may result in new health care priorities for the elderly and, ideally, decisions to pay for these services through a combination of personal funds, insurance, and government funding.

We will have to reach a wide range of audiences such as elderly patients, their families, long-term care administrators, insurance companies, and the federal government. We will need a different message for each of them but all our messages should reiterate the same theme: continuity of care for the frail elderly.

We can use several methods to change society's attitudes toward care for the frail elderly. For example, advertising that focuses on both the needs of the elderly and available services could be targeted to large audiences. Or on a person-to-person basis, a health professional can explain to an elderly person who needs care (and/or a family) why a service is recommended. Other effective ways to change societal attitudes about care for the aged might include open houses at nursing homes or "trade shows" which feature the types of services available in local long-term care facilities. Pamphlets, journals, and newspaper articles can increase consumer interest and knowledge regarding available sources of quality care. Insurance companies and the federal government respond most readily to research reports and articles, and the federal government frequently makes its decisions based on testimony presented at hearings. Whatever the method of communication, society's priorities must change. Our population is aging and the frail elderly will reach even greater proportions as those aged 65 years and over become an even higher percentage of the total population.

Reward for Service in Gerontology

Why do health professionals in gerontological care persist in the face of a disinterested society? Why do they worry about changing the curriculum when there is already so much to be taught? Why do nursing faculty learn new skills and create new knowledge in gerontology when they too could stay uninformed like the rest of society? Because caregivers enter their profession to meet needs. That in itself is the internal reward. Perhaps they hope that when they are old and ill, someone will care for them as they cared for others. Perhaps health professionals know that quality of life is important because they have seen so much pain and misery. Perhaps they hope that they are helping to move society to value the old and accept responsibility for those who are dependent and ill. This too is part of the reward for those who serve and care for the elderly.

There are also external rewards that help health professionals in their move to excellence in gerontology. Funding, for example, opens up opportunities for teaching, research, and practice. In turn, new job opportunities and new knowledge increase individual and university visibility, as well as a sense of pride in one's work and institutions. There are also the rewards that come from programs such as The Robert Wood Johnson Foundation Teaching Nursing Home Program which brought individuals and institutions national recognition. Those who were involved in the program were rewarded with the knowledge that the models created through the program are likely to affect a large part of society.

Preliminary findings from the University of Utah Robert Wood Johnson Foundation Project, for example, indicate that the patients and the nursing home team were rewarded for their participation. During the grant period at the nursing home, there were fewer falls, infections, emergency room visits, and hospitalizations. Clinical collaborations between physicians, nurses, and pharmacists greatly increased. The team reported an esprit de corps that promoted professional and personal growth—sufficient rewards to sustain commitment to values.[10]

Summary

The needs of the frail elderly are great but society has as yet to make their care a major priority. Societal attitudes can be changed through education and through a wide range of marketing and communications strategies. In the meantime, health professionals must continue to prepare themselves and their students for the care of elderly patients. The public must learn that these services are available and that they are of value. The rewards at present are sufficient to sustain such an effort, but health professionals alone cannot change the values of society. Academics and the larger society must make a concentrated effort to respond to the needs of the fastest growing segment of our population.

REFERENCES

1. Williams, TF. Geriatrics: The fruition of the clinician reconsidered. *The Gerontologist* 1986; 26(4), 345–349.
2. Donnelly, D. *Team: Theory and practice of team ministry.* New York: Praulist Press, 1977.
3. Ibid.
4. Feiger, SM, Schmitt, MJ. Collegiality in interdisciplinary health teams—Its measurement and its effects. *Social Science & Medicine* 1979; *13A*, 217–229.
5. American Association of Colleges of Nursing. *Essentials of college and university education for professional nursing.* Washington, DC: Author, 1986.
6. Watson, J. Nursing: Human science and human care, a theory of nursing. Norwalk, CT: Appleton-Century-Crofts, 1985.
7. Fox, WM. *Effective group problem solving.* San Francisco: Jossey-Bass, 1987.
8. Diers, D. *Research in nursing.* Philadelphia: J.B. Lippincott, 1979.
9. Hulbert, JM. (1985). Marketing: *A strategic perspective.* Katanoh, NY: Impact Publishing, 1985.
10. Cleary, M. Personal communication. Salt Lake City: University of Utah College of Nursing, 1987.

9

Ethics and Research in Teaching Nursing Homes

Neville Strumpf and Sr. Lucia Gamroth

A central task for the teaching nursing home was the creation of an atmosphere for quality care and research. Any research conducted in nursing homes, however, possesses special problems unique to institutionalized participants, including equity, freedom of consent, and the difficulties and dilemmas involved whenever subjects are physically frail or mentally infirm. The purpose of this discussion will be, first, to review the major ethical issues associated with research elderly persons, especially the problem of informed consent; and second, to describe how these matters are addressed in one teaching nursing home, namely the Benedictine Nursing Center (BNC) located in Mt. Angel, Oregon. The impact of these issues on all participants will be noted and questions will be raised for those engaged in similar affiliations.

Research on Elderly Subjects

The principles of ethical research are outlined in the Belmont Report to the National Commission for the Protection of Human Subjects of Biomedical and Behavioral Research.[1] Based on respect for persons, beneficence, and justice, these principles have special relevance for research with the aged.[2] The principle of respect for persons is derived from notions of self-determination and individualism. It requires that individuals be treated as autonomous agents and suggests that those with diminished capacity for autonomy require special protection. Beneficence requires a maximization of benefit and a minimization of harm. In taking seriously the caveat to "do no harm," the question, "Are the risks commensurate with the benefits?" must be answered satisfactorily. Finally, in the matter of justice, the burden of research needs to be distributed fairly in order to avoid any unfair burden because of social class, institutional location, or age. Researchers involving themselves with elderly persons, and the caretakers of those persons, must be concerned about the goals, purposes and moral justifications for specific investigations in aging; the analysis of risks and benefits for a potentially vulnerable population; the methods for equitable selection of subjects; and the determination of what constitutes fully or reasonably informed consent.

Since the establishment of institutional review committees in 1966, a trend to protect those research subjects deemed at "special risk" has been discernible.[3] Whether the elderly, by virtue of age, constitute a vulnerable group of potential research subjects requiring special protection is still being debated.[4] Cassell[5] argues that regulation cannot be relied upon to protect people from one another and furthermore, that such overprotectiveness has limited essential research of clinical problems of the frail elderly. Nevertheless, our experience with institutionalized elders suggests that three potential problem areas warrant special considerations before any research is undertaken.

1. *The nature of an institution*
   a) The facility becomes home, a place where the influence of those who work or reside there plays a significant role in determining participation and nonparticipation in activities, including research.
   b) The facility may contribute to dependency and acquiescence by residents regarding care.
   c) The facility is a public environment with attendant problems of maintenance of confidentiality.
2. *Characteristics typical of institutionalized elders*
   a) Many grow increasingly dependent and are, therefore, more vulnerable.
   b) Growing isolation and dependency may diminish the desire for autonomy in favor of security and human contact.
   c) Differing cognitive abilities, attitudes and values, including reluctance to offend those in authority, may alter decision making regarding participation in research.
   d) Physical, psychological, and social changes may decrease tolerance for what others define as "minimal" risks.
3. *Issues pertaining to investigators and their research*
   a) Research design may be inadequate in its attention to the special needs of older people, including appropriate risk/benefit analysis, selection of subjects, determination of competency, and consent procedures.

b) Conflicts may arise in situations where the caretaker is also the researcher or data collector.

c) Research situations can produce anxiety for elderly participants requiring special skill on the part of researchers or assistants in handling such stress.

d) Interventions may have unintended adverse consequences, especially with the elderly.

Institutional Review Procedures at the Benedictine Nursing Center

The nature of the institution, the characteristics of its elderly residents, and the research goals of investigators seeking subjects clearly affect decisions at the Benedictine Nursing Center regarding what research will be done and how it will be conducted. A 130-bed skilled nursing facility, the Center for years has been known for its innovative and dignified approaches to care of the elderly and the chronically disabled. As a "teaching nursing home" the facility became an even more desirable location for the conduct of research. Thus, a major challenge for the staff at the Center involved creation of a balance between the provision of excellent clinical care in a home-like atmosphere and the conduct of valid clinical research aimed at improvements in quality of care for the elderly. As the number of requests to conduct research increased, critical questions for the staff arose: Will the introduction of clinical research projects interfere with the staff's commitment to protect patient autonomy and dignity? How much interference with the daily routines of patients and staff can be tolerated? Who will ultimately control the processes associated with ongoing clinical investigations?

The Benedictine Nursing Center found it necessary to establish an institutional research committee to review and approve or disapprove proposed projects. A crucial first step for the committee is examination of the purpose of the project, especially for consistency with the Center's mission and determination of potential benefit to the residents. Careful review of the purpose usually clarifies appropriateness of the project for the setting. For example, interviews conducted at the Benedictine Nursing Center to aid in development of an instrument for assessment of functional abilities of elderly persons living at home probably are inappropriate for the setting. On the other hand, a well-designed study including interventions for wandering may be very relevant in settings where there are numerous wanderers.

Interventions which are part of the research protocol are carefully scrutinized, with special attention directed toward answering the following questions to the satisfaction of those in the facility:

1. Are instruments appropriate for the population and will they produce the data desired?
2. Are interventions appropriate to the setting?
3. How invasive are the interventions and how will they affect the resident physically, psychologically, and socially?
4. Do proposed benefits of the intervention outweigh the degree of risk or trauma to the resident or the resident's family? Consideration of the burden or stress to residents who have frequently been subjects in research projects is of special concern.
5. Will data adequately be controlled to assure confidentiality; how will findings be disseminated?
6. Is the project unique in its approach or have similar projects already been conducted at the Center?
7. Can the facility absorb such a research project at this time and still maintain the customary standards of care?

It is of special concern to the review committee to ascertain the degree of involvement by the staff in the project. If their workload is to be affected significantly, consent must be obtained from individual staff members, especially if participation means added responsibility for them. Time frame for the project is also considered. Sufficient time must be allocated to prepare staff, residents, and family members and to implement the protocol.

An additional critical step before approval of any research project is the interview of the researcher. This forms an integral part of the institutional review process and provides an opportunity for selected staff from the Center to obtain a sense of the investigator's "fit" with the philosophy of the agency and its personnel. During the interview of a potential investigator, it is helpful to ascertain his or her specific aims, perceptions of the impact on research participants, previous research with the elderly, and ability to work with the staff in a manner consistent with the stated beliefs of the agency. The interview also permits education of the staff regarding a particular project. If the project is to succeed, staff must be well-informed, for they are essential whenever something or someone is introduced into the system. When staff are well-informed, they feel part of the process of research and are more likely to facilitate the work of the entire project.

Types of issues which are addressed by the institutional research committee are illustrated by the following example. A proposal for a urinary incontinence study involving catheterization and cystometric testing on cognitively impaired females was submitted. Concern for the womens' perception of possible rape or attack was raised by the review committee. After much discussion of the benefit of correcting a reversible incontinence problem or detecting a pathological condition versus the risk of potential trauma, the committee concluded that the potential benefits of this study justified the intervention. Several approaches, however, were proposed to minimize the risk to patient subjects: (1) only patients with a reasonable potential for success would be considered for the study; (2) a clinical specialist, known to the patient, would accompany research staff during the procedure and serve as an advocate for the patient; (3) a procedure would not be completed on any patient who exhibited anxiety or fear.

Informed Consent of the Elderly

Of all the issues relevant to research with elderly subjects, none is more complex than assuring an individual's welfare through proper procedures for informed consent. Guidelines for the Protection of Human Subjects[6] refer to "informed consent" as "knowing consent of an individual or his legally authorized representative, so situated as to be able to exercise free power of choice without undue inducement or any element of force, fraud, deceit, duress or other form of constraint or coercion." In their excellent review of research with older human subjects, Kapp and Bigot[7] specify the requirements for informed consent:

1. A statement of the purposes of the research and the expected duration of the subject's participation, a description of the procedures to be followed, and identification of any procedures which are experimental.
2. A description of any reasonably forseeable risks or discomfort to the subject.
3. A description of any benefits to the subject or to others, which may reasonably be expected from the research.
4. A disclosure of appropriate alternative procedures or courses of treatment, if any, that might be advantageous to the subject.
5. A statement describing the extent, if any, to which confidentiality of records identifying the subject will be maintained.
6. An explanation for research involving more than minimal risk.
7. An explanation of whom to contact for answers to pertinent questions . . . and in the event of a research-related injury. . . .
8. A statement that participation is voluntary, refusal to participate will involve no penalty or loss of benefits . . . , and the subject may discontinue participation at any time without penalty or loss of benefits. . . .

The essential elements of valid consent are that it be both voluntary and informed.[8] In addition, the subject must be competent to consent; incompetent subjects should be used only in those circumstances when competent subjects cannot participate.[9] Berkowitz[10] argues that formulations regarding consent have shifted subtly since the Nuremberg Code of 1947, which explicitly stated that "voluntary consent of the human subject is absolutely essential." The word now is "informed," rather than "voluntary," although "informed" does not carry the weight of "voluntary." "Informed" indicates cognitive awareness; it does not necessarily reflect degree of willingness. Physical, psychological, and social changes may limit how well a subject is informed, and many characteristics of the institution, the elderly individual, or the investigator may be influential factors in the matter of obtaining or granting consent.

Consent Procedures at the Benedictine Nursing Center

The Center carefully weighs the above-mentioned complex issues in its procedures for monitoring informed consent. Recognition of the centrality of a resident's choice is a focal point when considering every research proposal. The specific needs, capacities, and desires of the resident come first. Staff perceive themselves as significant advocates for the residents, especially honoring their expressed wishes, followed by those of family members or other designated responsible persons. Again, several questions concerning the consent process must be answered to the satisfaction of the review committees:

1. What will be the specific procedures for determining the competency of an individual resident to give consent for the project?
2. Under what circumstances will consent by family or other designated persons be sought and how will consistency with the wishes of the resident, had he or she been able to give consent, be ascertained?
3. Is the consent form designed in such a way that it is understandable to the resident and/or responsible other and clearly provides for a choice to participate or to withdraw from the study without consequences?
4. Is appropriate provision made for those residents who are competent but do experience periods of transient confusion?
5. Is ample time allowed for the resident to comprehend fully the procedures for which he or she is granting consent.

Once the research is approved, and the project underway, it remains essential to observe closely the methods of sample selection. The pressure to obtain subjects can occasionally make researchers careless in obtaining full and voluntary consent from participants. It is important for staff to observe closely residents' responses while they are research subjects; some parts of the protocol may serve to upset or confuse residents or families, even when their consent was properly obtained.

Often residents and families do not realize what they have consented to or the ramifications of a specific research project; in these instances considerable effort to orient, support, and respect the wishes of residents and family members must be carried out, even when it means the loss of a subject from the study.

Two examples serve to highlight some of the problems of fully informed consent from an institutionalized older person or consenting family member.

In the first, a study of "wandering behaviors" was approved for the purpose of instrument development. Appropriate oral and written consents were obtained from participants. The investigation was already underway when the spouse of one of the study subjects requested information about changes in his wife's behavior as a result of the research. When the specific purpose of the study was reviewed with the husband, he became very agitated that his wife had been included in a study which was of no benefit to her personally. Considerable staff time was spent with the husband to help him deal with the misunderstanding; in the end, a decision was made to remove his wife from the study. It is obvious from this vignette that explanation during consent procedures of the purpose and proposed methods of investigation requires language which is understandable to patients and families. The need for researchers to ascertain individual interpretations of procedures and outcomes is also essential.

The second situation demonstrates the inherent problems with consent obtained from a relative by telephone. Over a two-week period, the wife of one of the Center residents was contacted to give consent for her husband to participate in an incontinence study and to be part of a film on the teaching nursing home being made at the BNC. In addition, the wife was asked in a third telephone call if she could be visited at home by a graduate nursing student affiliated with the Center. On the day the wife was to be visited at home, she arrived at the Center extremely confused about the numerous requests and consents and unsure who had called for what. Again, the lessons for researchers are obvious ones: It takes time to obtain a fully informed consent; face-to-face encounters are more effective than consents obtained by telephone; and coordination at the Center of simultaneous projects involving the same resident is crucial.

Implications for Practice

Several researchers point out the problems of truly informed consent with the elderly. Stanley et al.[11] showed that the elderly demonstrated significantly poorer comprehension of consent information. Riecken and Ravich[12] found that few medically dependent research subjects at four Veterans Administration Hospitals had a good understanding of the research in which they were participating and 28% were unaware at all of their participation, in spite of the fact that they had signed consent forms. In two studies in a teaching nursing home, Hoffman et al.[13] found the consent process extremely time consuming, often taking at least one-half hour and requiring follow-up visits. Refusals were related to invasiveness of procedures (venipuncture, catheterization), feeling like a "guinea pig," fearing that abnormalities might be detected or that complications could occur, apathy regarding study goals or unwillingness to be inconvenienced. Some would consent verbally but were unwilling to sign anything.

Several of these investigators conclude that consent procedures for the elderly need simple cognitive screening procedures to identify persons unable to participate in common health care decisions[14]; clearly and simply written consent forms; provision by the investigator for explanations consistently reported; and continuous reassessment of the subject's understanding.[15] It may also be useful to consider obtaining the consent in more than one interview and to establish a role within the institution for a "consent auditor".[16] In the case of transient confusion or fluctuating awareness, individuals may still be capable of giving informed consent, but it is crucial that the research procedures and the consent process are closely linked. For those unable to give consent, it is important to remember that consents given by proxy (institutional representatives or family members, especially in the absence of an advanced directive) may not be in the best interests of the patient or resident. In one study of informed consent, of the 55 proxies who believed that the patient would refuse consent, 17 (31%) nevertheless gave consent, in apparent opposition to the patient's wishes.[17]

In reviewing the appropriateness of a particular investigation, the protocols for the study, and the consent procedures, it must be kept in mind that adherence to rigid guidelines may be excessively paternalistic and furthermore, may reduce the very research needed to improve clinical practice. As Cassel[18] points out, "Some kinds of special protection may be more burdensome than participation in the research would be. . . . We need to develop guidelines that will protect subjects from exploitation, but not rob them of personal choice and an opportunity to participate in society." The hazards of paternalistic behavior toward the elderly are well known: deprivation of decisional autonomy, stigmatization, and elimination of possible benefits, both direct and indirect, which might accrue from participation in the research, including increased contact with others, added attention, and a break in routine.

Many elderly subjects might actually welcome the chance to make a contribution; thus, the need exists to consider ways "to promote the creative and free involvement of geriatric patients in the research process".[19]

Conclusion

We must not deprive ourselves and the elderly of valuable insight gained through clinically significant and beneficial research, by employment of overly protective research procedures. On the other hand, moral imperatives exist which require a careful examination of the type of research to be conducted consensually, and the subjects to be researched. In "Ethical Considerations in Gerontological Nursing Research," Davis[20] reminds us that "The ethics of any research situation reside in the researcher. To the extent researchers understand and take seriously the ethics of informed consent, to the extent they respect the personhood of older adults, many of the dilemmas that arise will be solved ethically." It is through the partnership created by academicians, clinicians, residents, family members, and others that an ethically-based research program of mutual benefit to all can go forward. Still before us is the demanding task of considering our ethical responsibilities in conducting research we believe to be significant and obtaining a maximum degree of informed and voluntary participation. Efforts such as the ones described here demonstrate how teaching nursing homes can help define and articulate the many issues associated with conducting research and obtaining consent with institutionalized elders.

REFERENCES

1. National Commission for the Protection of Human Subjects of Biomedical and Behavioral Research. *The Belmont Report: Ethical principles and guidelines for the protection of human subjects of research.* Washington, DC: National Institute of Health; 1979.
2. Reich WT. Ethical issues related to research involving elderly subjects. *Gerontologist* 1978; *18*(4): 326–337.
3. Makarushka JL, McDonald RD. Informed consent, research and geriatric patients: The responsibility of institutional review committees. *Gerontologist* 1979; *19*(1): 61–66.
4. Ratzan RM. Being old makes you different: The ethics of research with elderly subjects. *Hastings Cent Rep* 1980; *10*(11): 32–42.
5. Cassel CK. Informed consent for research in geriatrics: History and concepts. *J Am Geriatr Soc* 1987; 35: 542–544.
6. National Commission, 1979.
7. Kapp MB. Bigot A. *Geriatrics and the law.* New York: Springer Pub. Co., 1985; 175–176.

8. Ibid.
9. Annas G., Glantz, L., & Katz, B. *Informed consent to human experimentation: The subject's dilemma.* Cambridge, MA: Ballinger. 1977.
10. Berkowitz S. Informed consent, research and the elderly. *Gerontologist* 1978; *18*(3): 237–243.
11. Stanley B., Guido J, Stanley M, Shortell D. The elderly patient and informed consent: Empirical findings. *J Am Med Assoc* 1984; *248*(3): 344–348.
12. Riecken HW, Ravich R. Informed consent to biomedical research in veterans administration hospitals. *J Am Med Assoc* 1982; *252*(10): 1302–1306.
13. Hoffman PB, Marron KR, Fillit H, Libow LS. Obtaining informed consent in the teaching nursing home. *J Am Geriatr Soc* 1983; 31: 565–569.
14. Tymchuk AJ, Ouslander JG, Rader N. Informing the elderly: A comparison of four methods. *J Am Geriatr Soc* 1986; 34(11): 818–822.
15. Riecken HW, Ravich R., op. cit.
16. Ratzan RM., op. cit.
17. Warren J, Sobal J, Tenney J, et al. Informed consent by proxy. *N Eng J Med* 1986; *315*(18): 1124–1128.
18. Cassel C K. Research in nursing homes: Ethical issues. *J Am Geriatr Soc* 1985; *33*(11): 795–799.
19. Makarushka, JL, McDonald RD., op. cit.
20. Davis A. Ethical considerations in gerontological nursing research. *Geriatr Nurs* 2(4) 269–272.

10

Trade-offs in Evaluating the Effectiveness of Nursing Home Care

Peter W. Shaughnessy and Andrew M. Kramer

INTRODUCTION

In this chapter, our ongoing evaluation of the Robert Wood Johnson Foundation's Teaching Nursing Home Program is used to review issues and tradeoffs entailed in evaluation research in the long-term care field. The intent is to discuss several issues by illustrating them in the context of the teaching nursing home evaluation study, thereafter selecting and elaborating on certain key points as relevant considerations in long-term care evaluation research in general. The final section involves considerations introduced by virtue of affiliations of operational health care programs with academic institutions.

EVOLUTION OF THE EVALUATION STUDY OF THE TEACHING NURSING HOME PROGRAM

Background

Despite widespread agreement that serious quality of care and quality of life problems exist in nursing homes in the United States, consensus has

The background work for this paper was in part supported by grant Nos. 6439 and 18-P-98417/01 from the Robert Wood Johnson Foundation and Health Care Financing Administration, Department of Health and Human Services, respectively.

not emerged on the specific remedies for these problems. Several approaches to improve the quality of care and quality of life for nursing home residents are currently under consideration or exist in experimental stages in various locations throughout the country. The Teaching Nursing Home Program (TNHP) of the Robert Wood Johnson Foundation (RWJF) is one such approach. The University of Colorado evaluation study of the TNHP, cofunded by RWJF and the Health Care Financing Administration (HCFA), began in November, 1983. The TNHP demonstration was completed in mid-1987, with the evaluation study scheduled for completion about one year later.

From the outset, the TNHP demonstration was targeted at determining whether the approach could improve the quality of care provided to nursing home patients, and, to some extent, whether the approach is cost-effective. In view of the possibility that only certain practices or program attributes might be effective or cost-effective, the evaluation was structured to determine whether there were selected or essential features of the program which would merit further consideration. At this writing, the design and data collection stages of the evaluation study are nearly complete, although the final analyses have not yet commenced.

In considering the effectiveness of a program aimed at enhancing the quality of care provided to nursing home residents, a key decision rests with the selection of measures of effectiveness. Initially, the major intent of the evaluation study was to assess the program's clinical outcomes. This is, the extent to which the affiliation between schools of nursing and nursing homes directly benefitted patients was most pertinent to the evaluation.

Even with the relative dearth of well-established and thoroughly researched patient outcome measures in the long-term care field, the conceptual appeal of using outcomes as indicators of the effectiveness of nursing home care cannot be denied. At the same time, if the TNHP were found to enhance patient outcomes, then the means by which it did so, i.e., the service regimens and treatment patterns, would be important to ascertain. Given the state of development of outcome measurement in the long-term care field, exclusive reliance on patient outcomes must be considered unduly narrow for comprehensive evaluation. This reliance would be problematic, especially if enhanced outcomes were a long-term effect of the program, i.e., occurred only several years after the program was in place. Such a phenomenon could not be detected by monitoring outcomes during the first several years of the program's existence, but might potentially be detectable in a shorter-run analysis of changes and improvements in the provision of services to nursing home patients. Consequently, striking a balance between process and outcome measures of quality in evaluating the TNHP was judged appropriate and necessary.

In assessing effectiveness of a program such as the TNHP, offsetting costs as well as confounding factors were considered. Thus, issues related to the cost of potentially improved effectiveness and, to the extent possible, the replicability of such effectiveness in other (similar) settings must be addressed. With respect to replicability, the evaluation study was designed to control as well as possible for factors or covariates which might uniquely influence measures of effectiveness at the TNHP sites relative to comparison sites. One of the most important sets of confounding factors is subsumed under the general category of case mix. Since the study involves patients from Teaching Nursing Homes (TNHs) and comparison sites, it was desirable that the TNH and comparison patients be as similar as possible. The selection process for the comparison sites, to be discussed shortly, was structured with this objective in mind. Nonetheless, analytic methods were also designed to further compensate for case mix differences in view of the likelihood that the sampling and selection procedures would not be totally adequate for selecting similar TNH and comparison patients. Further, case mix changes over time would first be analyzed as a possible program effect. Thereafter, case mix indicators will be assessed as potential confounding factors to adjust for in examining effectiveness.

From the outset, the five primary questions of concern on the evaluation study have been:

1. Did case mix characteristics of the patient population served by nursing homes participating in a TNHP change after the affiliation was established?
2. Is the program capable of enhancing outcomes, especially discharge to independent living and avoidance of hospitalization, for patients in TNHs relative to patients in nursing homes with no funded teaching affiliation?
3. Does the program result in improved delivery of services and care to specific types of patients in TNHs relative to similar patients in nursing homes with no teaching affiliation?
4. Do the potential benefits of the TNHP approach outweigh any increased cost that may be attributable to the program?
5. What can we learn from the program that might:
   a. Improve nursing home care nationally?
   b. Be transported directly to other nursing homes?
   c. Be of value in health systems planning and regulation?
   d. Assist in restructuring reimbursement for nursing home care?
   e. Shape and strengthen mutually beneficial affiliations between nursing homes and schools of nursing?

In view of the relatively small number of facilities and even smaller number of geographic areas included in the demonstration, the evaluation was regarded as a feasibility study of the teaching nursing home approach. As such, it was primarily directed at assessing whether the approach was of potential value in improving the quality of care to patients in certain types of nursing homes. The patient population from which the TNHP residents were selected (e.g., largely patients in non-profit facilities, slightly above average in Medicare coverage, etc.) clearly does not encompass all nursing home patients in the United States, nor is it intended to do so.

As originally designed, the evaluation study was targeted at assessing effectiveness almost exclusively in terms of changes in patient status. As such, the primary effectiveness measures were to be patient-level outcome measures such as change in the presence and grade of decubitus ulcers, changes in functional abilities (e.g., dressing, bathing, incontinence), and changes in the presence and the severity of various types of infections (e.g., respiratory infections and urinary tract infections). In the research design stages of the evaluation, however, it was decided that outcome indicators based on individualized patient status measures were less appropriate from a policy perspective than broader utilization outcome measures such as discharge to independent living and avoidance of hospitalization. Concern surfaced that change in patient status attributable to the TNHP might be sufficiently marginal, nondetectable owing to measurement error, or sufficiently difficult to translate into cost, so as to render the evaluation of questionable utility in an overall policy context. Consequently, the evaluation was refocused on major utilization outcomes that translate more directly into cost (such as decreased hospitalization rates) or into clearly understood desirable outcomes (such as discharge to independent living). The study was therefore redesigned and continued to evolve under the general principle that policy relevant effects, treatments, and costs should receive primary attention.

As the study evolved, it became clear that measures of effectiveness based exclusively on utilization outcomes would also be inadequate, although a return to the highly specific indicators of patient status would not be appropriate. Two other types of effectiveness indicators are therefore being employed. First, an effort will be made to assess whether TNHs have significantly better treatment regimens or service programs (that are attributable to the TNHP) relative to comparison nursing homes. Second, for selected patient groupings changes in patient status will be monitored on a monthly basis for three months. In addition, changes in status between admission and discharge, and between admission and six months after admission, will be examined as outcome measures. In all, although not explicitly stated as a guiding principle at the outset, the study approach was refined by weighing the relative ability of competing methods in alternative substantive areas to shed practical light on quality questions. The five originally stated objectives persisted throughout the period of refining the study approach.

Comparative and Temporal Dimensions

The absence of adequate baseline data during the pre-TNHP period eliminated the possibility of a rigorous before/after or pre/post study. Further, a controlled study based on randomized trials was not possible. Therefore, the study approach involves two fundamental comparisons. First, TNHs are being contrasted with comparison nursing homes (CNHs). Second, despite the constraints preventing a rigorous pre/post study, certain attributes of the performance of TNHs during the demonstration period are being compared to similar attributes before the demonstration period in 1981 and 1982. Since it is necessary to collect data retrospectively for this second comparison, its utility is regarded as supplemental relative to the TNH/CNH comparison which will be based on prospectively gathered data. Certain comparisons of performance during the early and late stages of the TNHP will also be conducted in this context. Pre/post comparisons will be conducted for both TNHs and CNHs for selected utilization outcomes and case mix indicators. Trend data on CNHs will be useful in adjusting the pre/post TNHP differences for extant trends which were occurring over time independently of the TNHP, such as case mix changes owing to Medicare's Prospective Payment System for hospitals.

The most important comparisons will be between patient groups pooled across facilities. For example, patients from the eight TNHs selected for the primary data collection will be pooled for purposes of comparing outcomes, services, costs, and case mix with a group of CNH patients obtained by pooling patient-level data across the eight CNHS in which primary data are being collected. Analogously, patient-level data from the eight TNHs (or CNHs) will be pooled across facilities to compare basic casemix and certain utilization outcomes on a pre/post basis in TNHs (or CNHs).

Eight TNHs were selected from the total of 12 (one of the 11 schools of nursing was affiliated with two nursing homes) owing largely to budgetary constraints. The TNHs selected were those with the highest admission rates and/or shortest lengths of stay. This decision was made in view of the increased policy importance associated with shorter stay patients owing to earlier discharge from hospitals under PPS and to maximize the potential number of patients in the prospective admission sample to be discussed shortly. Initial consideration was given to selecting twice as many CNHs as TNHs, but the logistical burden of increasing the number of sites would have lowered the patient-level sample sizes. The CNHs were chosen to be as similar as possible to the TNHs in terms of their *group profile* on ownership, freestanding versus hospital-based affiliation, percentage of Medicare patients, percentage of Medicaid patients, length of stay, occupancy rate, urban/rural location, and state.

The TNHs and CNHs were not matched on a one-to-one basis owing to the difficulty of selecting a similar facility for each TNH in its own state. Nevertheless, state was used as a group profile variable because Medicaid reimbursement systems, regulatory practices (both of which vary at the state level), and other state-level factors can exert considerable influence on nursing home behavior. Since a one-to-one match was not possible for these variables, a profile match was the most reasonable way to proceed. The intent was to attempt to insure that the group of CNH patients was cared for in as similar an environment as possible to the group of TNH patients. The group profile variables were selected from a larger list of profile variables on the basis of: (1) their hypothesized influence on quality of care and/or costs; and (2) the extent to which data were available on each variable for potential CNHs. Several of the variables are in fact case mix surrogates (e.g., percent Medicare, percent Medicaid, length of stay, and freestanding versus hospital based), some are related to cost (ownership, freestanding versus hospital based, occupancy, and urban/rural location), and others were hypothesized to be related to significant behavioral incentives or patient care mores (urban/rural location and state).

In general, the facility-level matching procedure yielded a group of CNHs that were highly similar to the TNHs as a group (on the matching variables). The fact that the patient rather than the facility constitutes the primary unit of analysis in the study, however, required that the profiles of facility characteristics be examined at the patient level. Consequently, patient-level profiles for the facility characteristics were examined by disaggregating the facility-level variables to the patient level for the prospective samples employed to collect longitudinal patient-level data during the primary data collection period. Since the patent-level sample sizes were not the same for each facility, this yielded different mean values for the profile variables relative to those based on considering each facility equally (i.e., with equal weights).

The magnitude of these mean differences at the patient level (i.e., mean differences in facility characteristics considering the patient as the unit of analysis) was then taken into consideration in developing an algorithmic approach to determining sample sizes within each facility in order to minimize the overall facility profile differences between TNHs and CNHs at the patient level. Although the facility-level profile match and the algorithmic approach to specifying sample sizes at the facility level resulted in a substantial increase in similarities between TNH and CNH patients in terms of facility-level characteristics (over a random or less thorough selection of CNHs and sample sizes), significant and in some cases moderately substantial differences in facility-level characteristics still persisted in the patient-level samples, requiring covariate adjustment methods during data analysis.

Measures Involved

Comparisons involving case mix before and after the TNHP will be conducted using such indicators as Activities of Daily Living (ADLs such as feeding and bathing), indicators of cognitive/behavioral status (such as confusion/disorientation and wandering behavior), nursing/medical problems (including pressure sores, urinary tract infections, etc.), and demographic/social supports (such as age, marital status, and visitors). In addition to their use in comparing case mix before and after the TNHP, such variables will be employed as covariates in examining potential TNH/CNH differences in outcomes, costs, and service or process quality measures.

Service data will be used in two ways. First, descriptive information on services provided to specific types of patients (belonging to certain strata) will be used to compare TNH and CNH patients on the manner in which services are provided, including both the frequency of services provided as well as the providers of services. In this regard, information has been obtained on the frequency and provider of services such as timed voiding for incontinent patients, catheter irrigation for patients with indwelling catheters, and repositioning for bedfast patients. Second, for selected categories of services, process quality scores ranging between 0 and 100 will be calculated. The process quality scores will be calculated in a manner analogous to that described elsewhere.[8] Such scores are calculated to reflect increasing quality of service provision, up to 100% if services are provided to perfect accord with standards for care specified by clinical experts. Selected process quality scores will be calculated for individual services and groups of services provided to specific types of patients.

Outcome measures are divided into the categories of utilization outcomes and patient status outcomes. The more important utilization outcome indicators consist of discharge to the community (independent living) and inpatient hospitalizations. The costs associated with utilization outcomes are computed on the basis of average costs of the facility. For example, assuming a patient was discharged to independent living after four months, the total institutional cost would be calculated by adding the nursing home and hospital costs for the patient over the four-month period.

Patient status outcomes consist of actual changes in patient status indicators such as changes in ADLs, mobility, decubitus ulcer formation/resolution, and other selected chronic conditions. Outcome, cost, and process quality analyses will be conducted using different groups or strata of patients. The groups will be defined using three types of patient-level stratifying factors: (1) discharge status; (2) time period; and (3) case mix or patient status indicators. For example, all TNH and CNH patients who are ambulatory, independent in feeding, and have no severe mental/behavioral disorders (case mix stratifiers) will be compared in terms of length of stay until discharge to independent living. This patient group will include both patients who were discharged and those who were not discharged (no discharge status stratifier), and will pertain to the time from admission until either discharge or the end of the data collection period for the study (the time period stratifier).

As a second illustration, TNH and CNH patients will be compared using hospitalization rates during the six-month period following admission (the time period stratifier), not restricting the analyses to any particular types of patients in terms of patient status (i.e., no case mix stratifiers), and by restricting the analyses only to those patients who remain institutionalized over the entire six-month period (discharge status stratifier). In fact, in view of the data collected, the time period stratifier could be 6 months, 12 months, 18 month, or 24 months. In this illustration, the discharge status stratifier could also be removed, thereby adding patients who are discharged. Since hospitalization data were collected through community followup only for patients discharged within six months of admission, these analyses would be restricted to the first six-month period.

KEY ISSUES OFTEN INVOLVED IN TRADE-OFFS IN LONG-TERM CARE EVALUATION RESEARCH

Attributing Patient Outcomes to Treatment/Services

Not only is it difficult to predict the course of many long-term care problems and diseases, but it is also difficult to discern whether changes in patient or disease status are due to care provided rather than a host of other patient-specific or environmental factors. Regression or lack of progress in a patient recovering from surgery, for example, may be due to inadequate nursing home care or it may be due to factors such as: (1) a medical or postsurgical complication which has nothing to do with care received at the nursing home; (2) a functional limitation that impedes patient recovery; (3) an emotional or cognitive disorder; or (4) inadequate hospital or physician care. Taking into consideration the fact that most long-term care patients often have a number of problems affecting mobility, sensation, cognition, functioning, continence, affect, and motivation, it is clear that a range of factors and circumstances other than patient care can mitigate the progress or rate of progress associated with change in patient status. The challenge of measuring and attributing outcomes to actual care provided can be likened to the problem of detecting an electronic signal passing through a field of electromagnetic noise. A number of factors can influence how the signal is received, if at all, and the challenge in determining the proper attributes of the receiver is largely a function of obtaining information about the nature of both the signal and the background noise. This analogy pertains to the measurement of outcome quality or patient outcomes in that the outcome itself can be thought of as the signal, and the noise is the large number of other factors which can mitigate the signal or outcome. The measurement challenge is to develop practical methods of gauging changes in patient status over time, taking into consideration and collecting information on other background factors which can influence the actual measurement of such changes in patient status. These factors must then be compensated for analytically by virtue of covariate adjustment, randomization, and/or case selection.

The Need to Focus

Given the nature of the TNHP, a large number of options existed for structuring an evaluating study. Agreement on program objectives and study objectives was a necessary condition to designing the evaluation. In this case, the program objectives were quite clear and translated readily into evaluation goals. The relative priorities among competing evaluation goals, however, only became clear after considerable discussion and an assessment of the feasibility of collecting information of various types. One of the critical topics to consider at the outset was the breadth versus depth of the evaluation scope. The evaluation study could have been approached with the intent of examining a wide range of patient outcomes, costs, acute care utilizations, and staffing characteristics. The temptation to undertake a truly global evaluation of the TNHP was resisted since it would have resulted in sacrificing analytic depth for breadth. Thus, selected conditions, patient status indicators, utilization outcomes, and services were chosen in accord with the specific objectives of the TNHP. In this regard, various TNHs focused on incontinent patients, resolution of decubitus ulcers, use of psychoactive medications, etc. In view of the fact that the evaluation was designed to be a feasibility study, specific consideration of patients potentially impacted by such programs was emphasized in certain areas.

Case Mix and Outcome Quality

The case mix of a patient population refers to the overall health status of that population and in turn translates into the health care needs of the patients in the population. Thus, health status indicators for individual patients aggregated over all patients in the population of interest are used to measure case mix. In a rigorous sense, the term case mix refers to a group of patients and the term patient health status refers to an individual patient. Theoretically, the case mix of a group of patients refers to their service needs, independently of whether the services are actually being provided. Therefore, the presence, absence, or severity of problems such as malnutrition, confusion, incontinence, or impaired mobility determine the patient's needs. These then translate into more service-specific case mix indicators such as the number of patients in need of assistance with walking, assistance with toileting, etc. It is important to note, however, that these measures are different conceptually from the number of patients actually receiving walking assistance, toileting assistance, indwelling catheters, and the like, since the first measures patient needs and the second measures services received. In fact, the degree of concurrence between needs and services received is an indicator of the extent to which patient health care needs are satisfied and therefore yields process measures of quality.

Analogously, change in patient status or patient health care needs over time is an indicator of patient outcomes over that time period. Clearly, patient outcomes can have many dimensions, depending on the health status indicators of interest. Thus, for a given group of patients, case mix pertains to the health status or health service needs of the group at a given point in time. If attention is restricted to the same population group or cohort, change in health status or health service need indicators over time then refers to patient outcomes. As a result, precisely the same patient characteristics and measures can be used to reflect case mix at a point in time and patient outcomes over time. Further, since case mix indicators point to service needs, process measures of quality also are necessarily related to case mix indicators.

As the case mix of an institution changes, so too will its indicators of outcome quality. Since the TNHs may have been characterized by an increasing case mix intensity over time (according to the hypothesis that affiliation with schools of nursing might encourage the treatment of more complex cases), the individual indicators of patient outcomes for the evaluation study were partly selected with this in mind.

Measurement Issues and Time Periods

The above discussion highlights the fact that many commonalities exist in case mix and outcome measurement principles. In measuring case mix, patient status must be measured at a point in time, and in measuring outcomes, patient status must be measured again at a second point in time (and possibly a third, fourth, etc.) to assess change in patient status. Consequently, the added feature outcome measures bring about is the issue of empirically measuring change in patient status over time.

A variety of measurement scales exist to assess patient status. In assessing change in patient status over time in order to measure patient outcomes, the same variety of measurement approaches are available and even increased by virtue of the need to measure change. Depending on one's objectives, change can be measured in a variety of ways, including the actual magnitude of the change, the percentage of the change (if a continuous measure is used), the pattern of the change (i.e., improvement versus worsening), transitions in patient status from time point to time point, percent time in an improved or worsened state, etc. Even patterns such as improvement or worsening can be measured as dichotomies or using methods from the fields of time series analysis and stochastic processes.

An important issue in measuring outcomes relates to the number of time points involved. This topic is also tied to the length of the interval between data collection points. Ideally, a particular problem would be monitored continuously on a daily or an hourly basis, depending on the nature of the problem. However, this is usually not possible from a practical perspective. In addition to determining how many different time points should be entailed in assessing change in patient status over time, the validity and reliability of the patient status measured at a single point in time must be considered. For example, even in a measure so straightforward as blood pressure, there is inherent variability which must be taken into consideration. It is possible to measure blood pressure on ten consecutive days for an individual who is in the normal range and find that on one or two of those days his/her blood pressure is in a high range.

At the basis of the number of time points issue is the expected progression of the disease or patient status indicator of interest. Some diseases (e.g., rheumatoid arthritis) are relatively slow in progression, while others (e.g., infections) can follow a much more rapid course. This emphasizes the importance of the duration of each time interval as well as the total time interval of interest in assessing patient outcomes for a specific type of problem. Finally, at least in some instances, the functional form of disease progression (e.g., linear, exponential, growth model, etc.) also bears on the issue of outcome measurement. If the expected progression of a problem from one time point to another is linear (i.e., occurs at a constant rate of change), then the length and number of time intervals chosen is not as important as when the expected progression of the disease is exponential or logistic in nature.

The multidimensional nature of outcome measurement is also significant and as used here, refers to the many dimensions of health status. Thus far, this discussion has dealt with measuring single health status indicators (ADL, ADL index, severity of a problem such as decubitus ulcers, etc.), in a solitary or univariate sense. However, a patient is in fact a composite or constellation of health status indicators and, theoretically speaking, all signs ideally should be taken into consideration and measured simultaneously. Therefore, when conceptualizing a patient's health status at a given point in time, it is appropriate to think of that patient as a set or "vector" of observations or values of health status indicators, some measured as dichotomies, others measured on an ordinal scale, and others measured on a continuous scale. Considering change in patient status over time, one would then examine the difference in the various health status indicators between two time points for the elements of this vector. It would be ideal if we were able to somehow distill this entire vector of outcome indicators into a single measure capturing the total patient change over the time period of interest. In fact, this is not possible and we have to settle for approximations to it.

The foregoing discussion leads to the suggestion that it is unwise to use a single outcome scheme or paradigm in assessing the impact of long-term care programs on change in patient health status over time. Since few outcome measures in the long-term care field have been universally accepted or, more generally, are universally applicable, a logical way to proceed is to first select health status indicators that reflect patient problems the program under consideration is expected to deal with effectively. Then one can attempt to measure the extent or severity of such problems in accord with already accepted or reasonable measurement approaches, regardless of whether the approaches are dichotomous, ordinal, or continuous. In this regard, a multidimensional approach to outcome measurement using a number of different measures to assess outcomes or changes in status over time, is preferable to an unidimensional approach.

Cost in Resource Consumption

Although the evaluation of the TNHP focuses more strongly on effectiveness than cost, a more balanced treatment is presented here since other long-term care evaluation studies have placed equal or greater emphasis on cost. When possible, both the direct and indirect costs of care warrant consideration. The direct costs or care refer to costs incurred in treating the patient, such as costs associated with medications, staff time, and physical therapy. Indirect costs refer to costs incurred (or not incurred, i.e., a savings), usually outside the care environment of interest. For example, acute emergency care, inpatient hospital care, early discharge from a nursing home, substitution of outpatient for inpatient care, family time spent or not spent caring for the patient, and increases or decreases in SSI payments due to institutionalization (or its absence), all translate into costs, often termed indirect costs. The most important indirect costs in the TNHP evaluation were judged to be those related to inpatient hospitalization and early discharge. In fact, it was in these areas that the TNHP was hypothesized to be cost effective.

Direct patient care costs can be measured at the patient level or at the facility level. The standard approach to measuring facility level costs is to divide total facility costs for a given period of time by the number of patient days, thereby obtaining a unit cost based on the per day cost of providing care. This can be done for different cost centers, such as nursing salaries, administration, and property costs. Cost figures of this type can usually be obtained from audited Medicare and/or Medicaid cost reports at the facility level.

Patient-level direct costs, however, are more difficult to measure and typically require information on services consumed by patients, including the type of service, the provider, and the frequency with which the service was provided. If such data are available either through time and motion studies or are approximated using some form of patient log on a retrospective basis, estimated resources consumed by individual patients can be computed in dollars. An advantage of using patient-specific costs rests with the increase in degress of freedom for analytic purposes. In the TNHP evaluation, for example, with only 11 TNHs in the demonstration, only a small number of distinct observations for facility-level costs were possible. If patient-specific indirect costs or resource consumption indicators were used, however, the number of patients involved in the evaluation would then determine the number of observed cost values. This also addresses the problem of cost reporting differences among nursing homes that might result in noncomparable costs owing to differences in Medicaid policy from state to state.

Randomization versus Comparison Groups

The ideal method for assessing the impact of the TNHP outcomes would have entailed randomization. For example, at each location, patients would be assigned to a TNHP or a comparison facility not affiliated with the given nursing school. In this case, under the theoretical assumption of random assignment, the likelihood is small that the two patient cohorts would differ in terms of case mix characteristics (this is also a function of sample size, of course). Theoretically, the randomized design should also be blind in the sense that the providers at all participating facilities, including the TNHs, would not be aware of whether patients were assigned under this randomization process to their facility, or whether they were simply admitted using standard admission procedures.

Realistically, in many long-term care evaluations, a randomized design is not possible because: (1) the demonstration is already under way; or, more importantly, (2) the ethical and logistical barriers that would be encountered in implementing such a design are insurmountable. Nonetheless, an evaluation approach should be structured to approximate the merits of an experimental randomized design as closely as possible. In this regard, the most critical components of the design become those of controlling for patient (and nursing home) characteristics in assessing the impact of the TNHP in patient outcomes (costs). This clearly speaks to the need to assess outcomes for patients who received care under the TNHP relative to comparable patients who received care in the comparison facilities.

The question such a comparison would theoretically address is "what type of care would the TNHP patients have received if the TNHP were not in existence?" Hence, comparison facilities and comparison patients should be selected so as to insure, as well as possible, that treatment and comparison patients are similar in terms of health status and their care environment, exclusive of the presence of the nursing school affiliation. In fact, this sort of comparison design might also be thought of as approximating a before/after design.

Controlling for Nursing Home Characteristics

It would have been possible to obtain highly similar patients in the TNH and CNH cohorts if facility-level characteristics were disregarded.

However, if the facilities or care environments in which the two cohorts received care were radically different, one would not be comparing outcomes for patients who were in facilities similar to the TNHs prior to their affiliations with the schools of nursing. Hence, the goal of approximating the before-after design would not be attained. It was therefore necessary to select comparison facilities on the basis of key nursing home characteristics such as those enumerated previously. These characteristics were selected to be similar to those of the TNHs prior to the TNHP.

The issue of whether comparison facilities should be in the same geographic location is not always as straightforward. On the one hand, the opportunity to find CNHs similar to the TNHs is enhanced if comparison facilities can be selected with little or no geographic constraints. On the other hand, the geographic location of each TNH tends to serve as an inherent control for certain attenuating circumstances such as the stringency of Medicaid policy within a given state, state of local regulations that might influence nursing home care, etc. Thus, in the case of the TNHP evaluation, it appeared that the selection of comparison facilities should be restricted to the same states.

Another key issue in the selection of comparison facilities is the number of such facilities. Procedurally, it is easier to select facilities on a one-for-one basis, as was done in the TNHP evaluation. However, two factors can mitigate against this. First, patient-level analyses can at times require unusually stringent processes for selecting comparison patients, and therefore necessitate a large pool of patients from which to select different patient cohorts. Second, even after a relatively thorough process of attempting to select comparison facilities using a one-to-one matching procedure employing a number of facility characteristics, study and comparison groups can still differ in terms of average values for certain characteristics that might be important. In this regard, the notion of a "nuclear comparison group" would warrant investigation. The basic idea in constructing a nuclear comparison group is to select more than one comparison facility for each study facility, where the comparison facilities are deliberately selected so as to "encompass" the study facility in all relevant characteristics. For example, if only bed size and percentage of Medicare patients were used to select two CNHs per TNH, the CNHs would be selected in such a way that one comparison facility had more beds and the other fewer beds than the TNH of interest. Further, one would have a higher percentage of Medicare patients and the other a lower percentage of such patients than the TNH of interest. In this respect, each TNH can be regarded as the nucleus of a cell in which it is surrounded by CNHs (in terms of the attributes of interest). This analogy pertains best when a larger number of comparison facilities are used per study facility, although the basic rationale pertains with as few as two comparison sites.

COMMENTS ON COMPLEXITIES ADDED BY VIRTUE OF ACADEMIC AFFILIATIONS

The various topics or dimensions of evaluation research discussed above often require compromise in view of budgetary and time constraints, as well as program and evaluation objectives. In fact, a number of additional items and topics frequently are entailed, including selection of the case or unit of analysis, the extent to which an evaluation study should be informative and provide feedback to the program, and even a variety of logistical considerations that can result in tradeoffs such as reliability of measurement versus cooperative respondents. Any such study also has a variety of unique tradeoffs that must be taken into consideration.

In this regard, although unanimity existed on the fact that the study should focus on patient care and patient outcomes, emphasis on this objective to the relative exclusion of others entailed considerable deliberation. In particular, the TNHP had a number of other purposes related to affiliating nursing homes with schools of nursing. These dealt with:

1. Clinical leadership and expertise, role of nurse practitioners in nursing home care;
2. Inservice training;
3. Research activities;
4. Faculty appointments;
5. Continuing education opportunities;
6. Inpatient care linkages;
7. Clinical training for nursing students; and
8. Increased availability and retention of nursing personnel.

Although the study does not totally ignore these program objectives, the vast majority of time and effort is channeled toward attainment of primary objectives: assessment of the impact of the TNHP on patient care, patient care outcomes, and patient care costs. Data and information in several of these areas is being collected for descriptive purposes, however. Further, the TNHs and others associated with administering the TNHP have monitored such areas and reported pertinent information (including various chapters in this book). Regardless of the results of the empirical evaluation, it is important not to overlook information in these areas. The determination to target the empirical evaluation of the TNHP on patient outcomes of significant policy importance as reasonable in view of the potential for the TNHP to bring about changes in certain care practices, patient outcomes, and utilization outcomes such as hospitalization and early discharge. Such a focus is in keeping with the basic principle that an evaluation study should focus on the *raison d'etre* of health care, namely patient outcomes. In this regard, progam effectiveness ideally should be measured in terms of what happens to patients. Using this criterion, the three most intuitively appealing categories of effectiveness consist of patient status outcomes, utilization outcomes, and, to some extent, direct patient care (services), as discussed earlier.

Nevertheless, the academic affiliation that forms the basis for "treatment" under study gives rise to other surrogates or potential surrogates for effectiveness. Consider, for example, the issue of additional long-term care research or increased educational involvement on the part of a school of nursing in the long-term care field stimulated by virtue of a formal affiliation with a nursing home. While this does not guarantee immediate results in terms of changes in patient status, utilization outcomes, or even services provided, it has the potential to enhance all three over the course of time. As faculty become more involved in and cognizant of patient care needs and issues, new research projects and educational programs bear the potential to improve patient care. Unfortunately, however, the results of such efforts often only occur over the long run. These particular surrogates for patient care effectiveness, i.e., faculty-acquired research and curricula changes, are in a broad sense of bonafide value as long-term indicators. Changes in an augmentation to research and educational programs can exert considerable influences on the general patient care environment.

The main point is that while evaluation studies in the long-term care field must focus on certain objectives, the process of making tradeoffs and decisions regarding study characteristics and goals should not preclude a broad-based set of conclusions and final inferences. In the context of the TNHP, for example, this means first a review and summary of criteria used to select the focal points of research. Thereafter, final empirical results should be accompanied by the appropriate qualifiers in terms of areas excluded and factors omitted in view of selecting more relevant approaches. Where possible, reporting information obtained by or through others on matters related to other program goals and objectives should accompany conclusive data.

REFERENCES

1. Institute of Medicine, Committee on Nursing Home Regulation. *Improving the quality of care in nursing homes.* Washington, DC: National Academy Press; 1986.

2. Aiken L H, et al. Teaching nursing homes: Prospects for improving long-term care. *J. Am. Geriatr. Soc.* 1985; 33(3):196–201.
3. Glascock J. *The modified survey process—Traditional survey process evaluation project.* Seattle, Washington: The Hesperides Group; 1985.
4. Mathematica Policy Research, Inc. Evaluation of the state demonstrations in nursing home quality assurance processes. Final Report, Princeton, NJ.
5. Shaughnessy P W, Breed L D, Landes D P. Assessing the quality of care provided in rural swing-bed hospitals. *QRB* 1982; 8(5):12–20.
6. Weisfeld N. Accreditation, certification, and licensure of nursing home personnel: A discussion of issue and trends. Unpublished paper, 1984.

11

An Agenda
for the Year 2000

Linda H. Aiken

Health care in the United States is undergoing a period of unprecedented change due to social and demographic trends, changing patterns of disease, advances in science and medical technology, increasing physician supply and shortage of nurses, and economic pressures limiting the growth of health care expenditures. These factors will reshape the context in which health services will be delivered in the future with implications for the practice of professional nursing and the constellation of services available to the elderly.

DEMOGRAPHIC PROJECTIONS

Predicting the future is an imprecise science, particularly in the realm of medical care. One aspect of the future that seems certain is that more Americans will be living to older ages. Two factors substantially affect the future size and age distribution of the elderly population: the size of varying age cohorts and changing patterns of mortality. For example, based upon the number of infants born in the 1920s and 1930s, we can expect a modest growth in the total numbers of elderly until 2010. After that, however, the number of elderly will increase much faster as the post World War II "baby boomers" reach retirement age.

One out of every eight Americans is now 65 or older but by 2020, one in five Americans is expected to be 65 years of age or older. The fastest growing group will be those 85 years of age and older. Since all of those who will reach 65 by 2020 have already been born, we can be reasonably certain that the actual numbers of elderly will be *at least* as high as currently predicted. We cannot be as certain as to the denominator (people under 65), however, since we do not know what the birth rate will be in the future or whether major changes in immigration policy will affect the size of younger age groups. The size of the working age population is important in predicting the future of health services for the elderly since most of the financing of retirement income and health and social services for the elderly is derived from taxing the working age population.

We can be even less certain of how the size and age distribution of the elderly in the future might be affected by changing patterns of mortality. For example, because of changing patterns of mortality, people born today have an average life expectancy of 26 years longer than those born in 1900. The age-adjusted death rate in the U.S. has fallen by one-third just since 1950. Among the elderly, substantial reductions have occurred in deaths from 4 of the 5 leading causes of death. Only deaths from cancer continue to increase.

The impact of changing mortality patterns is illustrated by recent changes in death rates due to heart disease. Prior to 1960, deaths from heart disease had been rising at an alarming rate. Based on those trends, it was predicted that by 1984, some 163,000 people between the ages of 55 and 64 would die from heart disease. However, for reasons that we do not totally understand, death rates dropped and 60,000 fewer people in this age group died than had been predicted.

Changing mortality rates have stimulated a lively debate over future morbidity patterns among the elderly. It has been largely assumed that as life is extended the very old will experience increased morbidity and disability thus requiring more health and social services.[1] Fries[2] poses an alternative scenario suggesting that an increasing number of elderly persons will live long enough to reach their biological limits then die "natural deaths" using few health services prior to death. Researchers trying to unravel these competing views of the impact of an aging population on the health care system have made several interesting observations.

Contrary to popular belief, much of the elderly's use of health services is related to dying rather than aging. A very large proportion of total expenditures on the elderly are devoted to care in the last few months of life primarily due to large hospital expenditures at the end of life.[3] Many of those dying at older ages actually have less expensive deaths, some with few consequences to the health care system. The exception is the very old who tend to have heavy nursing home use in the final years of their lives.[4]

While there is much about the future that we do not know, it seems reasonably certain that there will be many more Americans who will be functionally dependent upon others than there are today even if the rate of disability does not increase with advancing age. Thus, different arrangements for organizing and financing long-term care will undoubtedly be required.

COST CONTAINMENT

National health expenditures continue to grow at a faster rate than growth of the general economy; health care is consuming a larger and larger share of the nation's wealth. In 1986, health spending rose to 10.9% of the Gross National Product (GNP), and health expenditures are expected to continue to grow more rapidly than the rest of the economy through the end of the century. By 2000, health care spending is expected to account for 15% of the GNP.[5]

Increased health expenditures affect all parts of the economy since employers bear a substantial share of the cost of health care. When health care costs increase, the prices of goods and services produced in the U.S. also increase, which contributes to making U.S. products less competitive in world markets. For example, the Chrysler Motor Company estimates that health insurance for its employees and retirees adds $500 to the cost of every new car it produces. Thus, businesses have become more aggressive in trying to restrain health expenditures.

The federal government has had a long standing interest in containing the rise in health care costs. A brief review of the federal budget will quickly indicate why. The federal deficit is at an all time high due to an excess of spending over revenues. Of course, the deficit can be eliminated at any time by increasing the government's revenue base through increased taxes. This has not been a popular option among politicians; therefore spending cuts have been the focus of most of the debate.

For all its complexity, the nearly $1 trillion federal budget can be broken down into four major components: national defense, assistance to the elderly, interest on the national debt; and other. Over 50% of federal domestic spending now goes to the elderly, primarily in three programs: Social Security, Medicare, and Medicaid. Together, national defense, programs primarily to assist the elderly, and interest already account for 75% of the total federal budget, and for 95% of future projected spending increases.[6] Thus, the major possibilities for slowing the growth of federal spending are the defense budget and programs for the elderly. Both defense and Social Security have had widespread political support to date which leaves health care programs for the elderly to bear the brunt of budget cuts. It is very likely that in the years to come the pressures to contain rising health care costs will focus more and more on the elderly since their care is so highly subsidized by government.

Two major strategies to reduce the growth of health expenditures currently dominant cost containment efforts. Both have substantial implications for nursing practice in general, and nursing services for the elderly in particular. The two are: controlling wages and prices; and reducing care. A third option which does not necessarily contribute to reducing the rate of growth of health expenditures but does help the federal government with its budget problems is increasing beneficiary cost sharing.[7] Of these strategies, reducing care holds the greatest promise of reducing the growth of health expenditures, and therefore increasingly will be pursued as an option in the years to come. It also presents the greatest risks of adverse affect on health outcomes.

So far, the major target for care reductions has been the hospital where per capita costs are the highest of any service setting in health care. Hospital admissions have been reduced substantially by a number of factors including advances in medical technology that now make it feasible to conduct many diagnostic and surgical procedures on an outpatient basis and cost containment efforts such as preadmission screening. Average length of stay for patients 65 years of age and older has declined by 20% since the introduction of Medicare's prospective payment system which reimburses hospitals by diagnosis not by length of stay (except for some unusual exceptions). As a result of both reduced admissions and declining length of stay, hospitals nationally provided 50 million fewer inpatient days in 1986 than in 1981.

A change as large as the recent reductions in hospital care inevitably affect other health care settings as well. Nursing homes, in particular, have experienced substantial changes in casemix. Hospitals are transferring patients to nursing homes earlier in the process of recovery and often when they are still acutely ill. The most recent data available on nursing home patients from the 1985 National Nursing Home Survey document both an increase in the proportion of nursing home residents 85 years of age and older and an increasingly dependent patient population.[8] Since all efforts to date to control rising hospital costs have failed, it is very likely that in the future the approach will be to use as little hospital care as possible. This translates into more rigorous hospital admission and length of stay criteria, and consequently increased pressures on nursing homes to accept patients with more complex medical and nursing care needs.

THE NATIONAL SHORTAGE OF NURSES

Despite very substantial increases in the supply of nurses over the past two decades, the nation continues to experience cyclical shortages of nurses. The current shortage is particularly perplexing because it occurred in the context of very large reductions in the number of hospitalized patients nationally. For example, since 1983, hospitals have closed more than 40,000 beds and average hospital occupancy rates dropped to 63% in 1986. Curiously, hospitals have dramatically increased the number of nurses employed at a time when there are fewer patients. Since the majority of nurses work in hospitals, changing hospital employment patterns have far reaching implications for the recruitment of nurses in other health care settings, particularly nursing homes.

The implications of the current nursing shortage for the future of nursing home care is unclear. Two primary factors appear to be responsible for the current shortage. One has to do with increased nursing care needs of hospitalized patients. With shorter average stays in hospitals and fewer discretionary admissions, patients on average need more nursing care. However, this alone does not explain why hospitals have employed so many nurses in the past several years.

An additional explanation is that the demand for nurses is excessive because their wages have been artificially depressed as a result of implicit wage controls. Nurses are very versatile in a hospital context. If their wages are depressed, it is more cost effective to have more of them and fewer aides and LPNs. Nurses can also substitute for nonnursing service personnel including ward clerks and couriers and for other health professionals such as physical therapists and social workers. Indeed, the evidence suggests that the current nursing shortage is due to broad scale substitution of nurses for nonnurses rather than an actual numerical shortage of nurses.

A solution to the nursing shortage, then, is to permit nurses' wages to rise enough to stop the substitution phenomenon. However, wage increases will be difficult to implement in the current cost containment environment. Increasing the supply of nurses is another intuitive solution. However, a 50% increase in the number of employed nurses over the past decade was not sufficient to meet the seemingly insatiable demand for nurses in hospitals. Moreover, it may not be possible to continue to expand the supply of new nurses. Enrollments in nursing schools have dropped by 26% since 1983. The attractiveness of nursing as a career seems to be declining relative to the other options available to todays young men and women.

If the current shortage of nurses persists, it will be very difficult to attract enough nurses to nursing home practice to implement needed change. While the current nursing shortage is often defined as a problem of hospitals, its solution is necessary to ensure that enough nurses will be available for long-term care settings.

ACQUIRED IMMUNODEFICIENCY SYNDROME (AIDS)

Changing patterns of hospital use and the aging of the population will continue to be major forces acting to reshape nursing homes and their respective roles in the health care system. Added to them is the emergence of acquired immunodeficiency syndrome (AIDS), a disease totally new to our society in the 1980s.

It is estimated that approximately 1.5 million Americans have been infected with the virus that causes AIDS. Because the disease has a long latency period, it is not yet clear what proportion of the infected population will eventually succumb to debilitating and/or fatal illnesses. Prospective cohort studies of infected persons have documented the progressive incidence of AIDS and associated medical conditions with each additional year after infection. Projections from these studies suggest that more than 30% of HIV-infected persons will develop AIDS within seven years of infection and another 40% or more will develop clinical HIV-related illnesses.[9]

The emergence of AIDS may be yet another powerful force shaping the future of nursing homes. The virus that causes AIDS, unlike many others, can cross the blood brain barrier resulting in severe neurological and cognitive impairment. There is increasing evidence that the central nervous system effects of HIV infection may begin very early in the course of disease.[10] At least mild cognitive impairment may be demonstrated in otherwise asymptomatic seropositive persons.[11] The incidence and clinical trajectory of cognitive impairment among persons infected with HIV is not yet known. Many suspect, however, that cognitive impairment will become an even greater source of disability for persons with AIDS whose lives have been extended by use of drugs such as AZT.

A high percentage of persons with AIDS live alone, at significant distances from nuclear family members, and many are at least moderately estranged from their families.[12] Thus, persons with AIDS with or without cognitive impairment, represent a potentially large group of people who are likely to require long-term nursing care in the future.

AN AGENDA FOR 2000

Nursing homes have experienced many problems over the past two decades balancing the competing demands of changing patient needs, constrained third party reimbursement, and the expectations of investors in what is a predominately for-profit enterprise. These problems have been well chronicled by Vladeck in *Unloving Care: The Nursing Home*

Tragedy.[13] The Teaching Nursing Home Program was designed to help nursing homes respond more effectively to the many and varied challenges of today and tomorrow. While much progress has been made in the nursing home sector over the past five years, a big agenda remains.

Developing Professional Nursing Practice in Nursing Homes

The changing patient case mix in nursing homes will increasingly require a shift in emphasis from custodial to therapeutic care, and a more effective interface between nursing homes and the rest of the health care system. In years past, nursing homes had few nurses, very uneven participation by physicians, and were isolated from the mainstream of American health care.[14] An underlying assumption of the Teaching Nursing Home Program was that the first step in a transition to a therapeutic environment was to attract and retain professional nurses in nursing homes.

Nursing homes are disadvantaged in some respect in terms of nurse recruitment. Salaries, on average, have remained below those offered by hospitals. And, the challenges of long-term care are poorly understood by many nurses. Thus, nursing homes will have to develop sone unique and attractive attributes to offset these negative perceptions and realities. Here, nursing homes have much to learn from the successes and failures of hospitals to attract and retain nurses. A large body of research is beginning to emerge on the attributes of hospitals that have been successful in retaining nurses even in the current hospital nursing shortage. Factors that correlate with higher satisfaction and lower turnover among hospital nurses include: salaried status rather than hourly pay; unit self-governance; effective support services; self-scheduling flexibility; support for education and research; a sense of personal autonomy and accountability fostered by the institution; and rejection of traditional nursing role limitations.[15,16]

Actually, nursing homes face less natural resistance in implementing many of the above elements of a professional nursing model than hospitals. For example, rejection of traditional nursing role limitations is one of the most important factors in improving nurse satisfaction. Nursing homes, because they have so little medical presence, have many more opportunities to encourage nurses to develop practice models which challenge their knowledge and expertise. One nurse respondent in the Kramer magnet hospital study followup had some good advice how to break out of traditional nurse role limitations: "Forgiveness is easier to get than permission!"

The Teaching Nursing Home Program has demonstrated that it is possible to develop an attractive climate for professional nurses in nursing homes. An important item on the agenda for the next decade is to put in place in every nursing home in the country those elements of professional practice that will be attractive enough to overcome the still prevalent biases among nurses against nursing home practice.

Nursing Home Reimbursement Reform

Reimbursement policies are extremely important in the U.S. health care system in shaping the realities of clinical care. In general, nursing homes are paid on the basis of a flat rate per patient per day with a differential paid for certain patients judged to have rehabilitation potential. Nursing homes located in a hospital are often paid at a higher rate than freestanding institutions even though there is not overwhelming evidence of substantially different levels of patient care needs in hospital-based nursing homes compared to freestanding homes.

The new Medicare prospective payment system encourages hospitals to discharge patients as soon as possible. The existing nursing home reimbursement system, however, has few incentives that would encourage nursing homes to admit the sickest patients. Some states are attempting to change the financial incentives for nursing homes by moving away from per diem standard rates to case mix adjusted rates.[17] If perfected, casemix adjusted rates have the potential to yield a more rational distribution of resources to institutions that are willing and able to care for a sicker patient population. A case mix based reimbursement system should help finance an enriched nurse staffing mix which would facilitate the development of professional nursing models of care in nursing homes.

The second area of reimbursement reform that should be included in nursing's agenda in the next decade is improved reimbursement for professional services in nursing homes including nurses. Where medical coverage is thin or uneven, nurses could undertake expanded responsibilities which have been shown to enhance patient outcomes and reduce unnecessary use of the hospital.[18] The major financial support for nurses now is imbedded in the per diem rate. When there is a third party payor, it is generally Medicaid. However, the savings achieved by reducing unnecessary use of hospitals generally are savings to Medicare not Medicaid, which currently finances most of the publically sponsored nursing care in nursing homes. Thus, there is a strong rationale for reforming Medicare Part B policies to reflect the contributions of the professional services provided by nurses, and to enhance the revenue streams to support expanded professional nursing models in nursing homes.

Third, high-priority should be placed on developing a more rational system for financing long-term care. By default, Medicaid has become an inadequate substitute for long-term care financing. Elderly persons needing nursing home care must improverish themselves and often their spouse as well. Medicaid reimbursement rates are often woefully inadequate to provide needed care. And the increasing demand on Medicaid for nursing home care threatens to undermine access to health care for the poor who also depend upon the Medicaid program for their health care. While there has been some recent growth in the availability of private long-term care insurance policies, less than 5% of Americans have any coverage for long-term care.[19] Moreover, most available policies are biased in favor of institutional care, benefits tend to be for a specified cash value unprotected against inflation (indemnity policies) and typically do not provide unlimited days of nursing home care for catastrophic illnesses.

Given the very high Federal deficit, it is unlikely that a new comprehensive publicly financed care benefit will emerge. However, it is possible that incremental changes will be made which together over the next decade will substantially improve financing for long-term care. Medicare's expansion to cover some catastrophic medical care costs may be the first incremental step towards long-term care.[20] The provisions of these incremental changes in reimbursement policy will be vital to the future of professional nursing in nursing homes, and nurses should take a proactive role in shaping new policies.

Educational Reforms

Most health professionals still receive very little exposure to geriatrics and gerontology. The vast number of new graduate nurses and physicians still have little or no interest in working in nursing homes.[21] Clearly, much more creative energy must be invested in the teaching-learning process as it relates to the health care of the elderly. An insufficient number of model nursing homes exist to convey to students the potentials of careers in nursing home practice. The Teaching Nursing Home Program has clearly demonstrated that is is feasible for nursing schools to "adopt" a nursing home and to help create an environment that will make a positive impression on students. Hopefully, more nursing schools will establish affiliations with nursing homes using the "blueprint" developed by the Teaching Nursing Home Program.

Also the placement of nursing home experiences in the curriculum is still without proper evaluation. Some educators believe that nursing homes are best for first clinical experiences because so many of the basic elements of nursing and medical practice are encountered. Others argue that the care needs of nursing home patients are too complex to be fully appreciated by beginning students. A continuing debate and objective evaluation is needed on all of the factors associated with the widespread implementation of more effective educational programs in geriatrics and gerontological nursing.

Research on Clinical Interventions and Health Services

To create a therapeutic focus in nursing homes, nurses need an armamentarium of clinical interventions with documented effectiveness. A high priority in the years ahead should be systematic evaluations of nursing interventions particularly for problems which commonly occur in long-term care settings and often result in progressive disability.

Likewise, additional research is needed on the organization of services for persons with long-term care needs. Much of the health services research on long-term care to date has served to question commonly held beliefs about the cost-savings potential of noninstitutional services such as adult day care and home care.[22] Community-based alternatives to nursing homes have often not proven to be substitutes for expensive institutional care but add-on services. We still know too little about how to target services to persons who would benefit most. Improving needs assessment techniques and learning to apply assessment techniques to target services for high-risk populations is an extremely important area of inquiry.

We know very little about how to best organize and deliver services for persons with AIDS. In general, persons with AIDS are significantly younger than nursing home residents. Should AIDS patients be integrated into existing long-term care facilities? If not, what kind of alternative would be more appropriate? How will health professionals be trained and deployed to care for the growing numbers of persons with AIDS and AIDS-related complex? What are the clinical nursing interventions that might delay disability and disfunction among persons with HIV related dementia? Health services research demonstrating and evaluating new nursing models of care for persons with AIDS is a high priority for nursing's future agenda in long-term care.

Conclusion

The provision of adequate health care for an aging population is a complex and multifaceted challenge. A number of different kinds of responses will ultimately be required. Teaching nursing homes offer promise as one strategy to help nursing homes respond to their rapidly changing environments. The Teaching Nursing Home Program has clearly underscored the need for developing and testing innovative strategies which together will provide the basis for a more rational and effective system of long-term care services for the nation.

References

1. Rice DP, Feldman JJ. Living longer in the United States: demographic changes and health needs of the elderly. *Milbank Mem Fund Q.* 1983; 61(3):362–96
2. Fries JF. Aging, natural death, and the compression of morbidity. *N Engl J Med* 1980; 303:130–35.
3. Lubitz J, Prihoda R. The use and costs of Medicare services in the last two years of life. *Health Care Financing Review* 1984; 5:117–31.
4. Roos NP, Montgomery P, Roos LL. Health care utilization in the years prior to death. *Milbank Mem Fund Q.* 1987; 65(2):231–254.
5. Health Care Financing Administration. National health expenditures, 1986–2000. *Health Care Financing Review* 1987; 8(4):1–36.
6. Etheredge L. The federal policy and budget context. *Building Affordable Long-Term Care Alternatives.* Washington, DC: National Governors' Association 1987.
7. Aiken LH Bays KD. The Medicare debate: Round one. *N Engl J Med.* 1984; 311(18):1196–1200.
8. Strahan G. *Nursing home characteristics: Preliminary data from the 1985 National Nursing Home Survey.* Hyattsville, MD: National Center for Health Statistics (Advance Data Number 131); 1987.
9. Allen JR, Curran JW. Prevention of AIDS and HIV infection: Needs and priorities for epidemiologic research. *Am J Public Health.* April, 1988; 78(4):381–386.
10. Navia BA, Price RW. The Acquired Immunodeficiency Syndrome dementia complex as the presenting or sole manifestation of human immunodeficiency virus infection. *Arch Neurol.* 1987; 44:65–69.
11. Grant I, Atkinson JH, Hesselink JR, Kennedy CJ, Richman DD, Spector SA, McCutchan JA. Evidence for early central nervous system involvement in the Acquired Immunodeficiency Syndrome (AIDS) and other human immunodeficiency virus (HIV) infections. *Ann Intern Med* 1987; 107:828–836.
12. Wolcott DL. Psychological aspects of Acquired Immune Deficiency Syndrome and the primary care physician. *Ann. Allergy* 1986; 57:95–102.
13. Vladeck BC. *Unloving Care: The Nursing Home Tragedy.* New York: Basic Books, 1980.
14. Aiken LH, Mezey MD, Lynaugh JE, Buck CR. Teaching Nursing Homes: Prospects for improving care. *J Am Geriatr Soc* 1985; 33:196–201.
15. McClure M, Poulin M, Sovie M. *Magnet Hospitals: Attraction and Retention of Professional Nurses.* Kansas City, MO: American Nurses Association, 1982.
16. Kramer M, Schmalenberg C. Magnet Hospitals. *Journ Nurs. Adm.* 1988; I:18(1):13–24; II 18(2):11–19.

17. Arling G, Nordquist RH, Brant BA Capitman JA. Nursing home case mix. *Medical Care* 1987; 25:9–20.
18. Kane RL, Hammer D, Byrnes N. Getting care to nursing home patients: a problem and a proposal. *Med Care* 1977; 15:174.
19. Institute of Medicine. *Toward a National Strategy for Care of the Elderly.* Washington, DC: National Academy of Science 1986.
20. Harrington C. Catastrophic health insurance: What is needed? *Nurs Outlook* 1987; 35:254–255.
21. Feldbaum EG, Feldbaum MB Caring for the elderly: Who dislikes it least? *J Health Polit Policy Law* 1981; 5(4):62.
22. Weissert W. Some reasons why it is so difficult to make community-based care cost-effective. *Health Serv. Res.* 1985; 20:423–433.

Index

DATE DUE

3-21-92			
MAR 1 7 1996			
APR 2 8 2000			
MAY 1 0 2001			
GAYLORD			PRINTED IN U.S.A.